Silence, Please!

The Little Book of Tinnitus

What You Need to Know About:

- Tinnitus
- Ringing in Ears
- Tinnitus Treatment
- Hearing Loss
- Tinnitus Miracle
- Tinnitus Causes
- And a Lot More ...

Dave Carmichael

Porch Dog Press

Printed in the United States of America

First Printing, 2012

ISBN-10: 1477437088

Porch Dog Press
3155 Rosenkranz Road
Tieton, WA 98947-9694

http://TheOldPorchDog.com

Acknowledgements

Love and thanks to my wife, Mary, who doubles as my EFL (Editor for Life). Her keen eye and working knowledge of the English language made this book far better than anything I could have done by myself. Moreover, her patience and good humor are evident every time I ask her to repeat something she has said to me. Some day I shall nominate her for sainthood.

Contents

Section 5: Related Diseases

Epilog

Addendum

Foreword

Iremember the moment it happened. I was standing by my mother's wood-burning kitchen stove, getting ready to go to bed on a cold Nebraska winter night.

Suddenly I felt what I called "dizzy." That's the word I used when I sat down on a high-backed kitchen chair and told my mother what was happening to me. Years later I would realize that I was not dizzy at all. I did not feel faint. The room was not spinning. There were no waves of nausea. But at age 10, I could come up with no other word to describe the strange feeling that out of nowhere had come over me.

More than anything I was frightened. What in the world was happening to me? My heart raced.

It was as if I was in a dream. Nothing seemed quite real. If I had been an adult, I might have said that it almost resembled an out-of-body experience, or that I was having a panic attack. My voice sounded strange to me, remote, and I seemed to have no control over what I was saying. My mother's voice seemed to be coming through a heavy veil I could not see. Then I noticed one other thing:

There was a high-pitched whine in both ears that seemed to be emanating from the middle of my head.

At this writing, I am 72 years old, and that whine is still there. It has been there constantly since that cold night in 1947. It is worse some days, some times of the year, but it has not increased its intensity over the years, and I have long since become accustomed to it. In fact, 99 percent of the time I am not aware it exists at all. I can hear it only when I concentrate on it, to see whether it is still there. It always is.

But I am no longer frightened. Part of that comes from simply having lived with that whine for so long. But the human face I attach to my lack of fear is that of an ear, nose and throat specialist I went to see in 1971 when I was 32 years old and was having a recurrence of those mysterious "dizzy" spells that plagued me as a child.

He was a young man. He wore his hair long and held it in place with a headband. I called him my "hippie" doctor, and it was from him that I heard the word "tinnitus" mentioned for the first time. I can quote you verbatim what he said to me after he had run me through several tests:

"There are some things we don't know much about, and we don't know what causes them. What you have is one of those things. But I do know this: whatever you have is not life-threatening."

I had always suspected as much. Nonetheless, to hear it from him lifted a great weight from my shoulders.

That weight was particularly heavy the first year and a half after my first "dizzy" spell at age 10. I was in sixth grade at that point, and I missed 23 days of school that year. Many of those days were spent in bed. Why the school allowed me to advance to the seventh grade I'm not quite sure.

I remember that at some point during that time I was able to take in a movie at our local small-town theater called "White Heat," starring James Cagney.

It was a big mistake.

Cagney played a psychopathic criminal who was devoted to his equally psychopathic mother. We learn later in the film that his father died in an insane asylum.

Cagney's character suffered from debilitating headaches and sometimes had fits of insane and violent rage. He went into a particularly violent rage when he learned in prison that his mother had been killed.

For a long time after I saw that movie I was convinced that my "dizzy" spells were somehow similar to what Cagney's character suffered, and that I was destined to go insane myself some day. Silly, I know, but I was 10 years old. The fear of insanity haunted me for months. I mentioned it to my mother once, and she said that I should not talk or think like that, for fear that it might come true. I never brought up the subject again. It was a scary time.

My mother took me to several doctors that first year. One suggested I needed more iron in my blood and prescribed a liquid iron supplement. It did nothing but upset my stomach, and I had to give it up. Another doctor thought I needed a tonsillectomy, and so my mother had it done. It made no difference.

A third doctor suggested to my mother, out of my presence, that I might have leukemia, which in those days was a death sentence. When Mom came out of the doctor's office and got into the car that I was waiting in with the neighbor lady who drove us to the office, she burst into tears.

And I screamed, "What is the matter with me!?"

The neighbor lady tried to comfort me. "You know how mothers are, honey, they cry over the littlest things. Don't you worry."

As it turned out, there wasn't anything to worry about, unless it was the state of medical technology in 1949.

By 2004, however, when I had my third episode of "dizzy" spells at the age of 65, the medical profession had made significant advances.

This time I had an electroencephalogram and an MRI of my brain. I had a number of blood tests. I wore a heart monitor for a couple of nights. I saw an ENT doctor and a neurologist. I tried acupuncture and chiropractic.

What were the results of all that? Nothing, except that they confirmed that my hippie doctor was right all those years before.

Maybe the medical profession hasn't progressed as far as I thought it had.

In any case, the neurologist I went to in 2004 also provided me with a memorable quote. Memorable, perhaps, because when showing me the MRI of my brain, he said I had a "young-looking brain." (It probably is a good idea for a doctor, when he has to admit he doesn't know what your problem is, to pay you a nice compliment instead. Sort of helps take the sting out of not knowing what ails you.)

So here was the neurologist's final piece of medical wisdom:

"Look at it this way: If this (the "dizzy" spells) only happens every 35 years, you won't ever have to worry about it again."

He was assuming, of course, that I won't live to be 100. He could be right, no doubt, but I'm going to do everything I can to prove him wrong.

Meanwhile, I decided some time back that my nearly lifelong history with tinnitus should be put to some use. I am a retired journalist, with more than 45 years of experience as a reporter and editor. And so it was natural, I suppose, that I would consider writing a book.

So that is what I have done. It is not a long book. You probably can get through it in one sitting. But I think it is a valuable book, and that you or someone you love with tinnitus will get a lot out of it. Here is my wish for you:

May the ringing in your ears cease forever, and may you have silence and peace. May the only ringing you hear be the bells in some far-off chapel.

Dave Carmichael, 2012

Section 1:
A Close Look at the Condition

What Is Tinnitus?

Imagine you are in a beautiful park with your closest friends. It is a bright day with wildflowers growing nearby, and you have burgers or steaks on the grill. You're enjoying a glass of iced tea and catching up on the intimate lives of your friends when you hear a bee. It is in your hair, right above your ear. You know this because you hear that annoying little buzz.

It is a subtle sound, but it grabs your attention and you can no longer focus on what your friends are saying. That quiet buzz continues despite your best attempts to move your head or swat the bee away. You stand up in the middle of your conversation and start shaking your head, desperate to get rid of the annoying buzz without getting stung. Your friends are laughing and trying to help, but you do not hear them. You can only focus on that noise and your attempts to get rid of it.

Even if you have not gone through this exact experience, you know what it is like to have a bee following you around with that annoying buzz. Bees are a wonderful part of the natural environment, but their noises do not belong inside your head. This is exactly what many people suffering with tinnitus experience with the noises that seem to implant themselves in their ears. They are simple, subtle or harmless noises, but they get very annoying if not downright painful when they refuse to go away.

Unfortunately, those suffering from tinnitus do not have the ability to jump up and shake their head around to swat the noise away. This book was written to give a deeper understanding of what tinnitus is and what sufferers go through trying to live with and/or get rid of the noises in their heads.

If you or someone you love has this condition, this book will help you understand all aspects of the affliction, from getting diagnosed and figuring out what is causing the noise to learning effective measures to make the noise more bearable.

Understanding Tinnitus – Just the Basics

Many people think of tinnitus as nonstop ringing in the ears. That is a legitimate way to sum it up if you just want a very basic understanding of the condition, but that doesn't exactly explain what it really is or how it affects sufferers. If you want to go just a bit deeper, there are a few things to understand:

1. Tinnitus involves a noise in the ears that is not necessarily always a ringing sound. Different sufferers will describe the noises that they hear in different ways, so it is not limited to ringing. For some it is more of a buzzing sound, while others say it is like having a leaky faucet in their ears.

2. The noise does not have to be consistent to be diagnosed as tinnitus. Some sufferers experience noise that comes and goes, while others experience an ongoing noise that never goes away.

3. Tinnitus does not have to affect both ears. It can be in one ear for some sufferers and both ears for others. In some cases, it can actually start in one ear and migrate into the other ear.

Tinnitus is basically noise in the ear that is not explained by the surrounding environment. It is like sitting at that picnic and hearing that bee buzz in your ear and having no way to make it stop. There are many variables that explain the way different people suffer with the condition. Some find the condition nearly unbearable and that it interferes with their daily lives, while others find it a mere annoyance.

Do You Have Tinnitus? Getting Started with Treatment

The first thing you have to do when noise starts disturbing your peace is see a medical professional. They will review your medical history and ask questions regarding your health, lifestyle, and any medications you might be taking. They will also look at your ears and ask for a detailed explanation of what the noises sound like.

The goal is to verify that the noise is not being caused by a larger medical condition or by medication that you might be taking. You will begin the journey to discover what is causing the noise and what you can do to make it as bearable as possible. You may never be able to completely get rid of the noise, but you can lessen the extent to which it interferes with your daily life.

What Are the Sounds of Tinnitus?

If you could line up 100 people suffering from tinnitus and ask them to describe the sounds they hear, you might doubt that they all suffer from the same condition after hearing their answers. Ask the same people whether their sounds seem to come from their ears or somewhere in their head, and you might be even more confused. Although there are some sounds that are routinely reported from tinnitus sufferers, the noise can be a bit different from one person to the next.

One person might describe her noise as a glass shattering on a kitchen floor over and over while someone else describes the subtle sound of a rushing river in the distance. The most simplistic definition of tinnitus is ringing in the ears, but it doesn't have to sound like ringing. It isn't always the same volume, either.

The noises of tinnitus vary because the causes of the condition vary. The sound is coming from a given source within the body, and that source will determine the type of sound produced.

For example, someone hearing noise because they have high blood pressure would naturally hear a different noise than someone with pulsatile tinnitus. The first person is hearing blood rush through an enlarged blood vessel, while the second person is hearing their own heartbeat.

There is a theory that many tinnitus sufferers are actually hearing signals being transferred between the brain and the rest of the body. The belief is that everyone hears small noises from their brain, but those sounds are normally covered up by the constant noise being picked up by the surrounding environment. Those who suffer from tinnitus could be picking up on those sounds because they are too loud to be masked naturally. If this is true, it could explain the wide variety of sounds heard by those with unverified causes of tinnitus.

It is more accurate to think of tinnitus as abnormal noise originating from inside the ear or head. Using a single sound such as "ringing" to describe the condition is a bit misleading. The most commonly reported sounds are:

- Ringing
- Buzzing
- Rushing water
- Clicking

The Sounds of Pulsatile Tinnitus

Pulsatile tinnitus is a special form of the disorder in which sufferers can hear their heart beating. The sounds heard by these sufferers tend to follow a rhythm or beat. The exact noise might be described differently from one sufferer to another, but they almost always report the noise moving to a particular rhythm. This is because the sound is being produced by the heart, which beats in rhythm.

Overlapping or Changing Sounds

The fact that tinnitus sufferers hear different noises from one another is interesting enough, but some sufferers hear multiple sounds. Many report that their condition started out with one noise and over time changed to another noise. There are even some cases where sufferers report hearing two or more noises all at once.

Overlapping sounds can be nearly impossible to live with and are more likely to interfere with daily life. If you were hearing a constant ringing, clicking and rushing water sound all at one time, would you be able to focus at work or listen to what your children are saying from across the room? It would be incredibly difficult, which is why those with overlapping sounds have an extremely challenging time having an ordinary life.

The Volume of Tinnitus

Volume is another area in which tinnitus sufferers tend to describe their sounds a bit differently. Most report a consistent sound of medium to low volume. Those that experience louder noises tend to have the most difficulty sleeping, concentrating, and participating in daily life. In some cases, sound masking will be attempted to at least take the volume of the sound down a bit. This does not work for every sufferer.

Many sufferers note that the volume goes up when they move their heads too quickly or stay in a noisy environment too long. The intensity of the sound goes up, sometimes to an unbearable level that forces a sufferer to avoid certain situations in daily life. Those who experience intensified sound when they move their heads might be forced to avoid intense exercise or activities that require falling, jumping, rolling, or other motions. This is a major interference in daily life.

What are Your Sounds?

If you are suffering from noises from the ear or head, it is important to see a doctor for an evaluation. A doctor can rule out any medical conditions that might be causing tinnitus as a symptom and might be able to help you identify the cause of the sound.

How Is Tinnitus Diagnosed?

The first step in treating your tinnitus is getting an official diagnosis. You might think you are suffering from tinnitus, but your doctor will want to rule out any larger medical conditions that may be causing the tinnitus. In some cases, you might be able to cure the tinnitus by treating the larger condition causing it. In other cases, the tinnitus may be completely unrelated to any other medical problem. The only way you will know that you definitely have tinnitus and what may be causing it is to see your doctor.

In most cases, a family doctor will refer you to an ear specialist, sometimes called an otologist or an ENT (for ear, nose and throat) doctor. The ear specialist will know more about tinnitus and will be able to start the process of diagnosis so you can be treated and hopefully start to feel better.

Phase One: Medical History

The first thing you will do is give your doctor a complete medical history so he or she has the information needed to start the diagnostic process. You should bring all medications that you take on a routine basis to the initial appointment and be ready to answer detailed questions regarding your health and lifestyle. You should be ready to describe the noise you are hearing and give an average of how long you have been experiencing that noise.

Some questions might seem completely unrelated to your tinnitus, but answer them honestly and be patient with this initial phase of diagnosis. Something as simple as smoking could be a factor in the noises you are hearing. Past traumas to the head could also be factors, even if they were experienced many years in the past. Be very straightforward with your answers so you have the best possible chance at getting an accurate diagnosis and finding the cause of your condition.

Phase Two: Testing

The next step is to go through testing so the specialist can verify that you do in fact have tinnitus and start the exploration for the cause of the noise. If you are working with a specialist experienced in tinnitus diagnosis and treatment, he should be able to give you a rundown of potential causes and determine which tests to deliver based on information already collected up to this point. You will be able to ask questions prior to undergoing any testing.

The first test most doctors will give is a simple x-ray. This is just to take a look inside the ear to see if there are any obstructions or malformations in the ear which may be causing the noise. If the problem is revealed, you might not need to go through any further testing. If nothing unusual is seen in the x-ray, you could move on to a CT scan or an MRI. This gives a more advanced look inside the ear to make sure there are no problems with the structure of the ear that could be causing the noise.

Whether the cause of your tinnitus is found in that first round of testing or not, you may be put through an audiogram to determine whether you suffer any loss of hearing. Many people experience tinnitus along with a loss of hearing, and the source of the hearing loss can be traced back as the source of the tinnitus as well. Even if there is another cause for the tinnitus, it is important to know if you are living with reduced hearing capacity.

Some doctors may request evoked response audiometry in some cases. This is an advanced diagnostic tool that uses a computer to scan the ear to look for any malfunctioning that could contribute to or cause the noise being experienced. This is typically not required if the cause of the tinnitus is found through more basic testing.

Through these tests, the cause of the tinnitus might or might not be discovered. Some people never know what is causing their ear noise, while others are able to clearly put their finger on a cause. The good news is a doctor can officially give the diagnosis of tinnitus even without a clear explanation of the cause.

Phase Three: Visiting the Dentist

This phase may not apply to you, but you should know about it just in case. Some cases of tinnitus can stem from problems with the jaw. An ear specialist may ask you to see a dentist experienced in these conditions just to rule out or verify jaw problems. You may work with the ear specialist and/or the dentist if a jaw problem is diagnosed.

Phase Four: Exploring Tinnitus

There are further tests that can be used either as an extended form of the diagnosis process, or as an exploration process to help tinnitus sufferers find treatment options for their condition. These tests are designed to match the tone and volume of the noises being heard so the doctor can hear what is being experienced. Different types of noises can tip the doctor off to the potential causes for the tinnitus, which can either validate a suspected cause or help narrow down the options for treatment.

Once it is clear that tinnitus is being experienced, you may go through even further testing to see whether the condition responds to masking. This simply means that you can use other noises to mask the noise being presented in the ear. For some, this type of treatment is very effective, but it doesn't work well for everyone.

The amount of masking you have to undergo to manage your tinnitus depends on your condition and how your ears respond to the masking. This is something that might not be explored in every case, but you can ask questions regarding the process and possibility of using it in the long term to manage the noise if it is used for your condition.

Putting It All Together

This seems like a long process that will drag on forever, but it actually goes rather quickly once you get into the process. Once you meet with your doctor and get the referral to the appropriate specialist, you will go through initial testing and should be given a diagnosis rather quickly. You might not know exactly what is causing the noise that fast, but you should at least be able to get the diagnosis and get suggestions on further steps to try to identify a cause.

Not everyone knows what is causing their tinnitus. Sometimes it takes a lot of testing to find the cause, and in the end you often just have the best guess or assumption of one specialist rather than a clear and proven cause. This does not mean you cannot move on to start treating your tinnitus. Once you know that this is clearly a case of tinnitus, you will be ready to start finding ways to bring some relief into your life.

Start the Process NOW

Many people suffer with tinnitus for a long time before they decide to see a doctor for an official diagnosis. The sooner you start the process, the faster you can start finding relief. Don't make yourself suffer any more than you have to. If you are hearing noise in your ear that comes and goes or doesn't seem to ever go away, you need to see your doctor and move toward a diagnosis. Get help so you can get better.

Tinnitus: The Long and Short of It

About 50 million Americans experience tinnitus, according to the American Tinnitus Association. That is a shocking figure, but only an estimated 16 million of those tinnitus sufferers will go in for medical treatment. Further, only 3 million or fewer will be permanently disabled by the condition. There are a few types of tinnitus that could be differentiated, but the most basic separation is between short- and long-term tinnitus. Although both are the same basic problem, they can be caused by different things and affect the lives of sufferers in different ways.

Short-Term Tinnitus

Short-term tinnitus can last for a few minutes, hours or days. It may come and go during that time or it may be a consistent annoyance. It is typically brought on by a short-term burst of extremely loud noise or some type of trauma to the head or ear. The sounds associated with this disorder are the same as the long-term disorder. Different people experience it in different ways, from a buzzing or hissing sound to a pounding or throbbing pulsation.

What makes short-term tinnitus different from the long-term version of the condition is the fact that it does go away within a reasonable amount of time. The long-term condition can last years. In some cases, it will lead to permanent damage or hearing loss. Those lucky to be afflicted with a short-term condition do experience complete relief of their symptoms within a few weeks, and it often goes away in much less time.

That doesn't mean a short-term condition is any less annoying or less difficult to handle. The noise can be extreme and can interfere with sleep. It also could affect the sufferer's ability to concentrate and carry on conversations while it is present.

In most cases, treatment involves using background noise to lessen the annoyance of the noises. Since it goes away fairly quickly, further treatment is usually not necessary.

Long-Term Tinnitus

Long-term tinnitus does not go away in a matter of minutes, days or weeks. It may be present off and on over a period of years, or it may be a consistent problem that never goes away. This is the more severe form of the condition, and it can affect the lives of sufferers in a very negative way.

If you have suffered from tinnitus, you know how irritating it can be to hear those noises in your head on a consistent basis. If you have never suffered from the condition, close your eyes and start humming. Don't hum a tune, but just one flat note that goes on and on. Keep making this noise for a few moments, and then imagine trying to carry on a conversation with a co-worker while the noise continues in your mind. Consider trying to focus on your work or watching a television show with that sound in the background of your mind at all times.

You probably see how that would become bothersome and even confusing. Now, consider trying to lie down in a dark room to sleep with that noise in your mind. This is where the real interference in life comes into play. Tinnitus can keep people up and limit the amount of sleep they are able to get each night. Sleep deprivation makes it even harder for them to focus at work and hold conversations, which makes daily life incredibly difficult to endure.

Treatment for long-term tinnitus typically involves some form of therapy. Sufferers have to learn how to deal with the interference in their life and how to cope with the noise day after day. There are also sound machines that may be used to take the volume of the sound down or bring temporary relief. Many sufferers are also able to turn up the background noise in order to drown out the sounds they are hearing in their mind.

Long-term tinnitus can come with hearing loss, which complicates the treatment and how sufferers learn to live with their conditions.

One thing that needs to be clear is that short- and long-term tinnitus can be caused by a one-time injury or blast of noise. It is not true that long-term conditions result from long-term exposures and short-term conditions result from a one-time exposure. Many sufferers are exposed to one loud burst of noise and completely lose hearing and suffer from tinnitus long term.

Tinnitus, Hearing Loss, Vertigo – What Are the Differences?

What are you suffering from? From tinnitus, or from vertigo? Do you have hearing loss? Do you understand what all three of these terms mean and how these conditions are different from one another? If you are unsure, you are among the millions of other people who sometimes use these terms interchangeably even though they mean very different things. Even if you think you understand what makes these three conditions different from each other, read through this chapter. You may find that there is more differentiating the terms than you realize.

What Is Tinnitus?

When you hear sounds that are not being produced by the environment outside of your body, you are suffering from tinnitus. Tinnitus can come with hearing loss, but hearing loss is a not a direct part of the condition. Any time you hear noises that others are not hearing and that are not coming from the outside environment, you are suffering from tinnitus whether you have hearing loss or not.

Tinnitus is often produced by your own body, such as in the case of damage in the inner ear or blocked ear drums. The sound may also be produced by restricted arteries in the body, or some other internal conditions. Even though these sounds are produced by your own body, they are diagnosed to be tinnitus because you should not be hearing your own internal functioning. In many cases, the sounds are unexplainable and the causes of tinnitus are unknown.

In very rare cases, the sounds of tinnitus can be heard by others around the sufferer. It is heard coming from the sufferer's body, rather than from the surrounding environment. If that person were not around, others would not hear the sound. Some sufferers in these rare cases may believe they are not experiencing tinnitus because others can hear the noise as well, but if it is originating from inside their own body and not the environment, it is tinnitus.

Tinnitus can affect one or both ears. It can last a lifetime or just a few seconds. The sounds can vary just as much as the causes.

What Is Hearing Loss?

Hearing loss is a lapse of hearing ability regardless of what other symptoms may be present. Some people experience tinnitus and hearing loss together, while others experience just one or the other. Many people with hearing loss do experience tinnitus, but the conditions are separate afflictions and do not always come together.

Tinnitus does **not** cause hearing loss. Think of them as two separate conditions that often come together for some sufferers, but which do not have to be a package deal. This is one of the biggest misconceptions for people trying to understand what tinnitus is, and what it is not.

Hearing loss does not have to mean a complete loss of hearing. It can affect just one ear or it can affect both ears. Reduced hearing or a partial loss of hearing is considered hearing loss. For example, some tinnitus sufferers report difficulty hearing as a result of the noises in their ears. It is like trying to talk to someone while sitting in front of loud speakers blaring music. These sufferers are considered to be with hearing loss, even though they have not completely lost all ability to hear.

The loss of hearing when related to tinnitus does not have to be permanent. If the tinnitus goes away, then the reduced ability to hear can go away as well. For many sufferers of both hearing loss and tinnitus, the tinnitus is caused by the source of the hearing loss. In these cases, the tinnitus can be longer lived or never go away at all.

What Is Vertigo?

Stand completely still but imagine your head remaining in motion. This explains the sensation of vertigo in overly simplified terms. Even though no physical movement is being made, sufferers of vertigo feel as if they are off balance or somehow still in motion. This causes dizziness that can lead to stumbling or falling down in severe cases. If you have ever had severe head congestion and felt like your head was an aquarium and you were slightly off balance when walking or sitting and standing, you have some idea of what vertigo feels like.

There are three different forms of vertigo, with the difference being the sensation of movement. Some sufferers feel as if there is movement inside their heads, while others feel as if things are moving around them, and still others feel as if their bodies are in motion when they are standing still. It is very difficult to move around with vertigo, and some sufferers will fall down if they cannot sit down when hit with this sensation of movement.

Vertigo is often confused with tinnitus, even though dizziness and noise in the ears are two very different things. This may be because vertigo is caused by inner ear problems, just like tinnitus. Meniere's disease sufferers often experience both vertigo and tinnitus, which can make daily life incredibly difficult. Even when they are experienced together, it is important to distinguish them as two different conditions with different symptoms.

What's Your Poison?

Now that you have a better understanding of the differences between tinnitus, hearing loss and vertigo, it should be much easier to determine which condition or conditions you may be suffering. This should help when talking to your doctor about your symptoms, but be wary of diagnosing yourself based on these short descriptions. It is always best to see a doctor and explain your symptoms to get a professional opinion and perhaps some testing to be sure.

If you are suffering two or three of these conditions at the same time, it may be difficult to pick them apart and identify exactly what is going on. Professionals will be able to help you put names to what you are experiencing. They may also be able to determine whether these conditions are connected or caused by the same problem. From there, they can help you come up with effective treatments or at least methods of living with the conditions if they cannot be cured.

Section 2: Causes and Effects

Common Tinnitus Causes
and How to Avoid Them

One of the most effective ways to deal with tinnitus is to educate yourself about the most common tinnitus causes and learn how to protect yourself against them. This might not help if you are already suffering from the condition, but knowing what causes it can help you avoid situations that will make your condition worse.

Extreme or Prolonged Noise Exposure

The American Tinnitus Association lists loud noise as the most common of all tinnitus causes. This can be a one-time blast of very loud noise, or it can be repeated exposure to loud noise over time. Many people assume you have to routinely expose your ear to very loud noise in order to experience tinnitus, but that is not true.

Many sufferers go to a music concert, sit too close to the sound equipment and get tinnitus. Others do simple things like operating a leaf blower and experience tinnitus. If the sound is louder than the sound of traffic rushing by on a nearby highway or closer to the ear than that, you run the risk of ending up with tinnitus. Many of these cases will be short lived and the noise will stop after a few hours or days, but it is possible to permanently damage the ear with a one-time blast of super loud noise.

You can avoid this cause of tinnitus by controlling the noise level in your natural environment. For example:

- Listen to your music through a radio rather than ear buds, or at least control the volume pouring through those ear buds.
- Do not sit very close to sound equipment at events using sound systems. Wear ear muffs if you might be around high noise levels.

- Be careful with everyday tools, especially yard tools.

Head or Neck Trauma

The American Tinnitus association lists head and neck trauma as the second most common of all tinnitus causes. Any type of accident that affects the auditory system or the ability for the ear and brain to connect can cause tinnitus. This is especially true if the trauma damages the ear on a cellular level. There are tiny hairs inside the ear that are crucial for the transportation of sound to the brain. If there is cellular damage that affects these hairs or the ability of the brain to connect with the ear, hearing problems and tinnitus can be the result.

The only way to prevent this cause of tinnitus is to protect your head and neck from trauma. This is common sense and is something almost everyone does anyway, but it might include wearing a helmet when bicycling or riding a motorcycle.

Hearing Loss

Partial or complete hearing loss in one or both ears is also one of the more common tinnitus causes. This cause can happen naturally with the aging process, or it can be accident or trauma-induced. Anything that might cause hearing loss can increase the risk of experiencing long-term tinnitus.

Excessive Ear Wax

This seems like an unlikely cause of tinnitus, but it really does happen to many people every year. Ear wax is designed to protect the inner ear from bacteria and irritation, but excess wax can become compacted inside the ear. This compaction is what leads to the noises associated with tinnitus.

The best thing you can do to avoid this cause of tinnitus is to go in for regular checkups and have the doctor look at your ears. He or she should alert you if there is too much wax and will clean it out as needed.

Medical Tinnitus Causes

There are many medical conditions that could potentially become tinnitus causes. Here are a few:
- Meniere's disease

- TMJ disorders
- Tumors
- High blood pressure

Any disorder that affects the neck, brain, ear, or blood vessels can become a cause of tinnitus. It is much harder to avoid these tinnitus causes, as they are actually symptoms of a larger problem. You typically have to learn ways to relieve the symptoms of the tinnitus along with other symptoms of the larger medical problem.

Unknown Tinnitus Causes

Unfortunately, many people never know what caused their tinnitus. Thousands of people experience short-term tinnitus without ever knowing the cause, but there can be an unknown cause for long-term tinnitus as well. In some cases, the tinnitus causes will eventually be discovered as other medical conditions are revealed, but in many cases it is a complete mystery. Of course, there is no way to prevent or control what you don't know is happening.

Stress, Anxiety, and Tinnitus

If you suffer from continuous tinnitus over a long period of time, you might eventually come to understand the connection between the noise in your ear and the stress keeping you up at night. Stress has not been proven to cause tinnitus, but many sufferers have reported an increase in volume or frequency of sound during times of intense stress. For some sufferers, even a minor amount of stress may aggravate their tinnitus.

Internal Stress Response

You know what happens on the outside when you get stressed out. You may be short-tempered and snap at those you love. You may withdraw from others and throw yourself into the process of solving the source of your stress. What you may not realize is that your body is reacting to the stress internally as well. When you experience something traumatic, your body could continue to register stress internally for many months or even years after the event.

The United States Department of Health and Human Services has identified the following internal responses common to the human body during and after a period of stress:

- Fatigue
- Insomnia
- Muscle Tremors/Twitches
- Breathing Problems
- High Blood Pressure
- Restricted Blood Vessels
- Fast Heartbeat
- Chest Pain
- Headaches
- Vision Problems
- Nausea
- Dizzy Spells
- Sweating/Chills

There are also a variety of mental reactions that have been noted, including the inability to focus and increased forgetfulness.

Extreme stress or a tragic situation could leave some people mentally absent, just trying to survive the experience.

Notice how many of these physical reactions to stress happen to be things proven to irritate or intensify tinnitus. For example, many tinnitus sufferers have difficulty sleeping. They find that the longer they are unable to sleep the worse their tinnitus becomes, and the worse the tinnitus becomes the harder it is to fall asleep. If long-term, consistent stress interferes with sleep at the same time, the tinnitus could potentially become worse over time.

High blood pressure and the restriction of blood vessels is another huge problem for those suffering from tinnitus. The sounds in the ear are often caused by the rush of blood inside the ear or head, and when the vessels become restricted the noise can become louder.

Anxiety Disorders and Tinnitus

In 2007, researchers at East Tennessee State University teamed up with the James H. Quillen Veterans Affairs Medical Center's Tinnitus Clinic to research the similarities between the body's reaction to tinnitus and the body's reaction to post-traumatic stress. They found that noise affects someone with tinnitus in much the same way it affects someone with post-traumatic stress disorder. Both conditions leave sufferers very sensitive to sound, and the sounds that would bother someone with one disorder would bother someone with the other.

They also found that more than 30% of their studied posttraumatic stress disorder patients also suffered from tinnitus. They recommended that audiologists take into consideration special treatment for those with both of these disorders, since the tinnitus and sensitivity to noise can be far more intense when PTSD is also a problem.

There have also been studies that found a connection between inner ear problems and stress. All of this research combined shows that there are connections between stress, anxiety and tinnitus. Anxiety disorders and anxiety-related conditions such as post-traumatic stress disorder affect the body much the same way that tinnitus affects the body.

Although there has not been a clear link proving that anxiety causes tinnitus or the other way around, it is clear that an increase of stress and anxiety can lead to enhanced tinnitus. Long-term stress can create louder tinnitus sounds over time or cause off-and-on tinnitus conditions to resurface. An anxiety attack could cause internal reactions that lead to instant intensification of tinnitus.

Can Stress or Anxiety Cause Tinnitus?

Research has not proven without a doubt that stress and anxiety can cause tinnitus, but there are many personal accounts of tinnitus sufferers who insist that their tinnitus is sometimes brought on by intense stress or an anxiety attack. In many cases, sufferers believed they had beaten tinnitus only to find that years later an injury or other intense stressor caused tinnitus sounds to return.

It is very clear that tinnitus can become intensified as a result of an anxiety attack or a stressful situation, but there are many people making the case for anxiety and stress as a cause of tinnitus in some cases. This may be a reflection of the well-researched fact that tinnitus and stress affect the body in a similar manner. Someone at risk for developing tinnitus may start hearing sounds as a result of the internal responses to stress.

Excitement and Tinnitus

When you hear the word "stress" you probably think of a negative sensation. Stress is what you feel when you lose your engagement ring down the kitchen sink, get fired from your job, or realize your toddler is missing in the middle of the grocery store. What you cannot forget is that stress can be a positive as well. The body responds to extreme excitement and anxiety over positive situations just as it would respond to negative stress.

An example of positive stress might be a child standing on stage at a school spelling bee waiting for his word. He is extremely anxious, yet he is excited because he was chosen out of many other children to be in that spelling bee. If he wins, he may be elated, but his body will react just as it would when in a negative stressful situation.

This means tinnitus sounds may become louder in these positive situations as well. When you go in for a job interview you may hear louder noise than usual as a result of anxiety, and that may make the interview more difficult to focus on. If you are hired on the spot and know your financial troubles are coming to an end, you will be excited and relieved, but the enhanced sound will likely continue because that excitement is registered as a state of stress internally.

What Can You Do?

There is no way to completely eliminate stress from your life. In order to live happily and feel fulfilled in your life, you need to set goals, interact with others, and participate in activities that you find enjoyable. Getting out there to live that fulfilled life will naturally bring along some periods of stress. It may even bring along an accident that leads to intense physical pain or a traumatic event that leads to post-traumatic stress disorder or intense prolonged anxiety.

What you can do is try to minimize the physical responses to stress listed in this chapter. Keep your blood pressure under control by exercising and following a healthy diet. When you are under stress, use the deep breathing exercises presented on pages 77-79 so you can control the immediate spike in blood pressure. If you are under a lot of stress on a daily basis, take time to meditate or do yoga. Make sure you are taking care of yourself so you can handle stress with a lower chance of increasing tinnitus sounds.

If there is any way you can avoid a stressful situation or take a source of stress out of your life, do it. It is not worth the risk that those sources of stress could lead to intensified tinnitus. If you need medication or therapy to control a more severe anxiety condition, then get the help you need. You may be surprised to find that it not only soothes the mind, but soothes the sounds in your ear or head as well.

Tinnitus and Sleep Deprivation

Which came first, the chicken or the egg? is one of the oldest riddles known to man. Why it has lasted so long is kind of a riddle itself. The fact is that neither the chicken nor the egg can exist without the other, so which came first is really kind of a pointless, even silly question at best. But that hasn't prevented people from debating it for centuries. If nothing else, it makes for an enjoyable way to while away a few minutes in idle, pseudo-intellectual discussion. Your answer to the question, if you come up with a serious one, probably has something to do with your religious or spiritual views.

Well, believe it or not, there is a very similar debate going on in relation to tinnitus, which is much more real and much more serious than chickens and eggs. The question is: Which comes first, tinnitus or sleep deprivation?

Many tinnitus sufferers also suffer from sleep deprivation, but which is the cause and which is the effect? Is the noise in the ear causing sufferers to lie awake, tossing and turning because the noise keeps them too alert to sleep? Or are a sleep disorder and the lack of sleep the cause of the noise in the ear?

Professional opinions make the case for each of these scenarios, but it is likely that the answer varies from one sufferer to another. Some people may have a sleep disorder that leads to tinnitus as a symptom or result of the sleep deprivation. For others, the noise in the ear may interfere with sleep and thus lead to sleep deprivation.

Tinnitus can be amplified by the lack of sleep, whether sleep deprivation is the cause of the tinnitus or not. Most sufferers find that the noise becomes louder when they are not getting the rest they need. Those suffering from occasional tinnitus often find that the noise starts up when they are stressed and not well rested.

The Starting Point

If the cause of your tinnitus has been verified by a medical professional as something other than the result of a sleep disorder, you can safely assume that your tinnitus came first with the sleep deprivation coming second. If the cause of your tinnitus has not been verified by a medical professional, you should start by visiting a doctor to discuss your symptoms.

Try to estimate the date or period of life when your tinnitus first became a problem, and then do the same for the date or period of life when you first started having sleep problems. You may be able to estimate which came first by noticing which became a problem first, but it still might not clear up the issue completely. By working with a medical professional you can come to a better understanding of what might be causing your tinnitus.

In some cases, it may not be clear what is causing the tinnitus or the sleep problems. You may be asked to go through a sleep study to rule out any other sleep disorders. From there, other possible causes of tinnitus can be explored. Whether the cause of the tinnitus is identified or not, you will have to learn methods of dealing with the noise in your ear when you lie down to sleep.

The Dangers of Sleep Deprivation

Some dangers of sleep deprivation are well known. You wake up feeling groggy, your head may hurt, and you have difficulty focusing on even the smallest tasks. You may need a steaming cup of coffee to wake up enough to drive to work or go about other tasks in your day.

Other dangers may not be so obvious. Studies have shown that people who suffer from sleep deprivation routinely are at higher risk for heart attacks and strokes. Your tinnitus might not be a health hazard in itself, but the sleep deprivation that comes along with it might be a danger to your life.

Getting the Sleep You Deserve

Not everyone is lucky enough to get rid of tinnitus quickly. If you are one of the unlucky ones, you might want to learn to deal with the noise so you can get more restful sleep. Start by setting up your bedroom for the best possible outcome every time you lie down. Make sure the room is quiet. Turn off the television to eliminate distractions from the flashing of light around the room. If you need background noise to help mask the noise in your ear, listen to a soundtrack with nature sounds, or open the bedroom window if outdoor sounds are soothing to you. But try not to use the television or radio. They can keep your brain alert and interfere with your ability to fall asleep.

You can also follow some basic lifestyle rules that will help you fall asleep:

- Avoid foods that cause physical discomfort or stomach upset.
- Make sure your room is very dark, even if you have to use blackout curtains on the windows.
- Keep a consistent and comfortable temperature inside your bedroom year around.
- Do not sleep during the day so you will be tired at bedtime.
- Go to bed at the same time every night and get up at the same time every morning, including weekends and days you do not have to get up early.
- Avoid exercise within a few hours of bedtime.
- Learn meditation and deep breathing exercises that can be used to calm the brain and body.

Note that these suggestions have nothing to do directly with your tinnitus. They are geared to ensuring your body is ready to sleep and your brain receives the proper signals that it is time to sleep. By ensuring your mind and body are relaxed and ready for sleep, you have to contend only with the noise in your ear when you put your head to the pillow.

One Last Tip

If you find that you get more and more irritated the longer you toss and turn, you might be keeping yourself awake longer just by trying too hard to fall asleep. If you cannot fall asleep within 20 to 30 minutes after going to bed, get up and do something you find relaxing. You might meditate, read a relaxing book, or sit in the dark and listen to soothing music while sipping a warm cup of herbal tea or milk. When you start to feel more relaxed, give sleep another try.

Even if you cannot fall asleep as soon as you might like, make sure that you still get up at your usual time the next morning. You might not feel well rested, but you will be even more tired and ready for sleep when bedtime rolls around again. Avoid sleeping during the day, especially after 3 p.m.

Remember the dangers of sleep deprivation. It is worth working consistently to get the sleep you need and deserve.

Why Does Tinnitus Cause Depression?

There are some lucky tinnitus sufferers who find the noise in their ears a bit annoying, but nothing serious enough to complain about. Then there are the unlucky sufferers who find themselves sitting up in the middle of the night, hands pressed to their ears and tears in their eyes. Fast-forward 12 hours to the middle of the afternoon, and you can often find these unlucky tinnitus sufferers half asleep at work trying to focus or curled up on the couch avoiding interaction with the rest of the world.

Rather than living life to the fullest, you might find yourself depressed as a result of your tinnitus. This can happen over a period of time if tinnitus is left untreated or if few methods of relieving the noise and pressure work for you. Some people can even become depressed rather quickly after the start of tinnitus because the noise is so unbearable it forces them to withdraw from their normal daily activities.

The Importance of Sleep

It is believed that a leading cause of depression in tinnitus sufferers is sleep deprivation. Many find that the noise in their ears intensifies at night. This is probably because the external noise dies down in the later hours, and there is a long period of near silence. The tinnitus noise might not actually become louder, but it *seems* more intense because there is not as much background noise for it to blend into or be masked by.

The human body needs sleep to function properly. When you rest, the brain has a chance to catch up on signals and messages that have been firing off rapidly throughout the day. Your muscles are given a chance to relax and recoup from the day's activity, and they might start to recover from any exercise sessions during the day. You should wake up feeling fresh and ready to face a new day, solve problems and overcome challenges.

When tinnitus keeps you from falling asleep until the wee hours of the morning or wakes you up every couple of hours throughout the night, it takes a toll on your body. You find yourself foggy headed and unable to concentrate at work. You snap at your children for no apparent reason. You might argue with your spouse or other loved ones because you are not thinking clearly and are unreasonable in your demands.

You might put your life in danger if you drive without being fully awake. As the lack of sleep crosses the line into complete deprivation, you can find yourself depressed and withdrawing from the life you would otherwise enjoy. This is your body getting into a defense mode. It is slowly shutting down and closing off to others because your tinnitus has made you sleep deprived and completely miserable.

Sleep deprivation should be dealt with as quickly as possible. It is believed to be a leading factor in the onset of depression, and if you are forced to drive or operate other equipment it could even become a threat to your life or the lives of others.

Communication, Tinnitus and Depression

Imagine yourself sitting in front of a fan on high speed, with the air blowing directly into one ear. Now imagine trying to have a conversation with someone sitting across the room. You cannot turn the fan off or decrease its speed. How easy do you think it would be to carry on that conversation?

This is the situation many tinnitus sufferers find themselves in every single day. Others speak to them, but the noise in their ears makes it extremely difficult to hear what anyone is saying and to form an intelligent response. Having telephone conversations can be even more difficult, especially if there is any type of background interference, which is frequently the case when talking on a cell phone in a public place.

This makes many tinnitus sufferers pull away from interactions with others. Communication problems presented by tinnitus interfere with their social lives, and become an easy path to depression. Humans are designed to socialize with one another. We are creatures of companionship. Without daily communications and the enjoyment of others, we naturally start to feel alone and isolated. That can lead to depression in most people.

Stress and Irritation

For some sufferers, the depression is caused by the simple irritation of the nonstop noise in the ear. It is not so much about the problems caused when communicating with others, but the simple fact that no matter what they do, they cannot turn off that noise. There is no on/off switch. They have no control whatsoever over this annoyance.

In cases of short-term tinnitus, the noise eventually goes away, and the victims are able to forget about it (at least for a while) and go on with their lives. Long-term sufferers, however, have to deal with the noise day in and day out. Thus, they often tend to slowly become more and more stressed until they end up depressed. The depression comes on simply as a result of stress and the nonstop feeling of having absolutely no control over their own bodies.

Dealing with Depression

It is easy to say, "You need to get your tinnitus under control in order to rule out depression." Many sufferers get confused when they hear that advice, because if they could get rid of tinnitus they would in a heartbeat. For many, it is not as easy as that little piece of advice makes it seem.

In some cases, you have to deal with depression as a symptom of tinnitus while working to relieve the tinnitus itself. Treating depression is not something you should blow off with the notion that it will one day go away when your tinnitus is cured. Start immediately by taking some simple actions to help relieve the depression while searching for that tinnitus cure:

- Get out for a walk or perform some other form of exercise. This does not have to be intense exercise. The goal is to get out of your home and take in some fresh air. Oftentimes, depression gets deeper and deeper the more you hide from the world. It is difficult to get yourself up and moving sometimes, but make the effort and you will be rewarded.

- Set goals and lay out clear steps to reach them. Focus on these goals so you have something to get out of bed for each day. Make the goals creative and exciting so you want to reach them.

- Learn deep breathing exercises that will increase oxygen supply to the brain and help wake you up. This can be very effective if you struggle to focus at work because of tinnitus and depression.

- If you believe you are sleep deprived, see the chapter in this book regarding sleep deprivation (page 29). Tips in that chapter help you get more restorative sleep so you are at least less deprived than you find yourself today. This can be a key to overcoming your depression.

- You may also want to talk with a medical professional if your depression continues long term. It is important to seek help if you start to have thoughts of harming yourself or others. There may be medication that can help you overcome your depression, or just talking with someone about your experience with tinnitus might help bring peace of mind.

Section 3:
A Widespread Problem

Who Is Affected by Tinnitus?

A long list of celebrities have, or are believed to have, tinnitus. When you listen to the stories of these celebrities, you find one thing most have in common: Many of them attribute their tinnitus to loud sound on movie sets or continuous exposure to loud music during concerts. Pete Townshend has been very open about his long-term tinnitus, and quite a few other musicians, comedians and actors have suffered from hearing loss, tinnitus, or a combination of the two.

This does not mean tinnitus is a condition that is exclusive to celebrities and rock stars. It is now estimated that at least 30 million Americans suffer from this disorder, with hundreds of thousands more reported in the U.K. Most countries of the world now recognize tinnitus and have patients suffering with the condition to some degree.

Because there are many different causes of tinnitus, this condition could affect virtually anyone alive today. For some, the noises present themselves early in life and stick around for the long term. For others, the noises come on suddenly and might go away within a couple of days, return off and on, or stick around for the long term. The type of noise presented and length of suffering depend on the cause of the tinnitus.

This is a condition that affects every sufferer in a different way, so there is no way to say what types of people it affects or what they go through while living with it. What you can do is break it down to particular categories of people who might be more vulnerable to attacks of tinnitus. This could be a genetic vulnerability for some, but for most it is a vulnerability created by lifestyle and surrounding environment.

Tinnitus in the Music World

People involved with amplified music could be at risk of developing tinnitus, simply because they frequently are exposed to loud noise. This exposure to loud noise is one of the leading causes of this condition, so certain music lovers and performers put themselves at heightened risk.

Even if you are not a celebrity and do not play in a band, you could still be at risk if you attend a lot of concerts or frequent social events where loud music is played. You can help protect yourself by staying away from speakers and other sources of loud sound as much as possible. Just being in a smaller setting with a loud noise vibrating around you can increase your chances of developing tinnitus.

Tinnitus in the Workplace

Some people can increase their chances of developing tinnitus just by going to work. Work environments that include loud noises from machinery or tools can be just as damaging to the ears as a loud concert hall. This is why many industries provide headsets to block out sound for employees working in high-volume environments.

If you work in an environment with loud noise, remember to protect your ears. Wear protective headgear, even if it doesn't look so hip. If someone you love works in such an environment, remind him or her to do the same.

Meniere's Disease

Meniere's is an inner ear disease associated with hearing loss and the loss of balance. Sufferers endure attacks during which they experience vertigo, tinnitus, fluctuating hearing loss, and sometimes nausea. Sufferers are known to lose their balance and fall from time to time as a result of dizziness created by the disease. Sufferers also experience tinnitus in most cases.

There are different theories about the causes of Meniere's, but it is believed to be a result of physical occurrences inside the ear. Experts now believe it might be caused by the fluid in the ear either creating pressure inside the ear or not draining properly.

What is known is that sufferers are prone to attacks of tinnitus along with vertigo.

Tinnitus and the Elderly

If you think you are safe from tinnitus because you are older now and well beyond your days of partying in clubs or attending rock concerts, you should be aware that you still aren't off the hook. Tinnitus is very common in the older population. This is simply a reflection of the fact that there are more causes of tinnitus besides loud music, and many of those causes are associated with aging.

For example, hardening of the arteries is common in many older people and can contribute to tinnitus. Also, many people experience hearing loss as they age, and in many cases that can come with long- or short-term tinnitus.

Ear Infections or Malfunctions

Anyone prone to ear infections will be at higher risk for developing tinnitus. Although some of the noises experienced by tinnitus sufferers are described as coming from the head, many sufferers hear the noise from within the ear. Inner ear damage, blockage, malfunction or infection can cause noise that is identified as tinnitus.

Inner ear problems that are effectively treated and cured could come with short-term tinnitus that goes away when the problem is cured. In other cases, repeat infections or short-term damage can lead to tinnitus that sticks around for the long term. It is not completely understood why some people continue to have tinnitus even after their infections, blockages or malfunctions are cured. It is likely that some damage to the ear remains even after the initial cause of the tinnitus is believed to be cured.

Those who experience injury to the ear could also be at high risk for developing tinnitus. In some cases tinnitus can develop months or years after the injury, while in other cases it sets in immediately.

In many cases, the causes of tinnitus are unknown. This means it can potentially affect anyone, and that includes you and the people you love. Everyone needs to be aware of this condition and its most common causes so they can protect themselves as much as possible. Even with awareness and protection, many people will develop tinnitus. There is no way to know for sure who will be affected and who will be spared.

Tinnitus in Children

Line up a hundred children and select 13 of them at random. According to the Center for Disease Control, this is about how many children will suffer from tinnitus or find themselves at heightened risk for tinnitus during their younger years. That number may seem high, because tinnitus is not a childhood disorder that is routinely discussed. The bad news is that many children suffer from tinnitus without getting a proper diagnosis or treatment. The good news is that most do not carry the disorder into adulthood.

Diagnosing Tinnitus in Children

It is believed that more children suffer from tinnitus than we know today. The problem is that children do not have the ability to detect problems, voice their suffering, and express what is wrong in the same manner as adults. It is believed that many children who suffer from tinnitus start to show symptoms at a young age, when they are unable to effectively communicate what they are experiencing.

Many children will believe that their noise is natural. It is how they have always experienced the world, so they do not realize that certain sounds are not coming from the natural environment around them. Some may assume that everyone else hears the world the same way.

This can make diagnosing tinnitus in children difficult. Because children might not complain of sounds and the inability to turn them off, parents often do not suspect tinnitus. Symptoms might be treated as problems in themselves.

An eventual diagnosis might be made as the child grows up and is able to describe the sounds he or she is hearing. Some younger children will send signs by pressing on their ears, digging into their ears or otherwise showing that there is something wrong with the ear. When hearing loss is detected or a child has trouble hearing because of the frequency of the noise, it is more likely that an adult will pick up on the problem and eventually the tinnitus will be diagnosed.

If a child has mild tinnitus that does not overwhelm and aggravate, the condition might go undiagnosed for a considerable time. If the child simply believes the noise is normal, she may never say anything about it to others. Hearing tests can reveal the problem in some cases, but for other children it might simply go undiagnosed.

Outgrowing Tinnitus

The American Academy of Otolaryngology has revealed that the majority of children suffering from tinnitus do not enter adulthood with the condition. This should give all parents of a child with tinnitus hope that their child will also be free from the suffering one day.

This is great news for children who believe unwelcome sounds are normal and never get the treatment they deserve. Whether they experience ongoing tinnitus that eventually goes away or their sounds come and go throughout childhood, most will be free from the disturbance before entering their adult years.

Treating Tinnitus in Children

If a physical problem is found in the inner ear, it usually can be treated efficiently. If the cause of the tinnitus is unknown, children are often forced to learn to live with the sound just as many adults have to learn to live with their tinnitus. If the sound is of high frequency or volume and does not go away, it can become a severe disturbance to a child. In some cases, it can prevent a child from doing a lot of the things she might otherwise enjoy, such as dancing to music or playing outdoors where other children are making noise.

For a child who also suffers hearing loss, a hearing aid will typically be used. The hearing aid will allow her to communicate with others and hear the world around her better, but it might also decrease the sounds presented from the tinnitus (hearing aids tend to mask the tinnitus sounds). The level to which the hearing aid improves tinnitus will vary from one child to another. There is no simple answer that cures the problem for all children.

In many cases, children can learn to use sound to mask the noise in their ears. Sound masking is used for adults as well, so it is nothing experimental or risky. Different types of background sound will work better for different children, so it might take a bit of trial and error to find the right masking solution for a given child. For some children, masking will not work at all, and other methods of soothing will need to be explored.

Children under Stress

Children who suffer from consistent tinnitus or very loud tinnitus go through all of the stress and aggravation that is common to adult sufferers. The problem is that most children do not have the coping skills to deal with this type of life disturbance. They can get frustrated when they cannot hear something or when they have trouble communicating with others, and that problem needs to be addressed quickly by parents. The following tips will help:

1. Have a medical professional explain to the child what tinnitus is. The parent should then follow through and talk to the child about the way he experiences the tinnitus. Children need to understand what is happening to them, and they need to know that they will likely outgrow the problem. Just having that understanding and the support of a parent can make it easier to cope with the emotional and mental aspects of the disorder.

2. Teach children the deep breathing exercises presented on pages 77-79, or have a child psychologist come up with similar exercises for the child. Children will deal with the stress of their condition much better if they know how to soothe and relax themselves.

3. Do everything possible to make sure the child receives adequate sleep. Tinnitus can be made worse by sleep deprivation, and sleep deprivation will make the emotional aspects more intense.

There is no way to ensure a child never experiences tinnitus. Parents just need to be aware of the condition so they can pick up on subtle cues that their small children may be hearing unnatural sounds.

Tinnitus in the Armed Forces

In the book *Noise and Military Service,* researchers examined the theory that hearing loss and cases of tinnitus in ex-servicemen and women were directly attributable to noise they were exposed to while in the military. The book explores the question of whether military personnel were suffering from tinnitus and hearing loss as a result of their service in the military, or just as a natural occurrence associated with aging.

The results of the researchers' study are quite interesting and shed a lot of light on the effects military service might have on the ear health of some servicemen and women:

1. Ex-military personnel over the age of 80 were likely to experience hearing loss or tinnitus regardless of whether they were exposed to loud noise during service. The study concluded that once the age of 80 is reached, everyone is equally likely to suffer from hearing loss or tinnitus regardless of events earlier in life.

2. Ex-military personnel at the age of 50 did show an increased chance of experiencing hearing loss or tinnitus if they were exposed to loud noise during service. This increased risk for military personnel is comparable to the increased risk that everyone runs when exposed to loud noises in everyday life.

The military risk also is equivalent to the risk that rock stars put themselves at when they play their music in small clubs or listen to their recordings through headphones in the studio. The noise can have a negative impact on the inner ear. Tinnitus and/or hearing loss can be the result.

Is This a Serious Problem Today?

The American Tinnitus Association estimates there has been an 18-percent increase in the number of military veterans requesting help with tinnitus and related problems since 2000. The association also lists tinnitus as the No. 1 medical condition suffered by veterans today. If this data is accurate, tinnitus clearly is a major problem for those serving in the armed forces.

Not all military personnel have the luxury of spending their service time behind a desk in a quiet environment. Many if not most soldiers are exposed to the noise of gunfire, heavy equipment or explosives. And the noise of firefights in actual warfare can be extremely intense.

It does make sense that those serving in the military would be at far more risk of suffering inner ear damage and hearing loss than the average civilian in the United States.

For soldiers, it's not a simple matter of staying away from the speakers at a rock concert. Military personnel have to worry about numerous sources of loud noise, and avoiding those loud noises is not possible in many situations. Some military environments are just plain unhealthy for the ears, and protective gear currently available is obviously not enough for many soldiers.

Duration of Tinnitus

The research in *Noise and Military Service* also revealed that many military sufferers would recover from their tinnitus or hearing defects within a month of the exposure to a loud noise. This refers to those who were exposed to one instance of loud noise and then allowed the time to fully recover with proper treatment. This gives some hope that many suffering from tinnitus will recover. Results were inconclusive on whether the noise could lead to recurring periods of tinnitus and/or relapsed hearing loss later in life.

The hope of recovering does not necessarily extend to those soldiers who are exposed to continuous noise while on the front lines of battle or in other field positions. Continuous exposure to loud noise does increase the risk of tinnitus dramatically, and many military personnel do suffer from permanent hearing loss or ongoing tinnitus as a result of noise levels in the field.

Protecting Your Hearing in the Military

It can be more difficult to protect hearing during military service than in other positions in life. Someone working on a construction crew or in a noisy factory will be offered a headset to block out a lot of the noise, but that is not always the case with a soldier in the military. There is no warning when a gun is going to be fired or a landmine is going to explode.

In some cases soldiers will need to listen as closely to their environment as possible to stay safe, so wearing noise-blocking headsets is more of a danger than a help. This leaves them at increased risk for hearing loss or tinnitus if there is an unexpected loud explosion or if they are caught up in a sudden firefight.

The military has set some standards to protect soldiers' hearing as much as possible in the field, but many experts believe a lot more needs to be done in this area. Although it is difficult to protect against all risks to hearing out in the field, some professionals argue that more technology could be developed to help soldiers protect their hearing in sensitive situations.

If more soldiers were aware of tinnitus and their heightened risk for developing it, they might be more inclined to go out of their way to protect their ears in every way possible.

The problem is that most military settings do not allow soldiers many options for protection. When a loud explosion goes off, a soldier's first concern is his survival. He is often unaware of the damage to his ears until later, when he is suffering from tinnitus and/or hearing loss.

Treating someone in the military for tinnitus is just like treating everyone else for tinnitus. In many cases, veterans simply have to learn to live with the condition once they are out of the service.

Rock 'n' Roll and Tinnitus

Although there are many acknowledged causes of tinnitus, rock 'n' roll still gets a lot of the blame for the prevalence of this condition. It has been estimated that as many as 50 million people around the world have suffered from tinnitus in the past or are suffering with it right now. Not all of these people are suffering because of their love of music, but for many of them music has a lot to do with the problem.

The main connection between rock 'n' roll and tinnitus is the volume of the music. Tinnitus is often caused by blasts of loud noise, and rock 'n' roll is best enjoyed at high volume. Tinnitus can result instantly from one loud blast of noise, such as the noise from a large speaker at a rock concert. Tinnitus can also be caused by continuous exposure to noise over time, such as the noise of music from headphones, ear buds or speakers in a bedroom or home.

When you think about these connections between rock 'n' roll and tinnitus, you see how a lot of rock lovers could potentially be at risk of developing the condition.

Tinnitus and the Musician

Musicians – especially rock musicians – are at great risk for developing tinnitus and suffering hearing loss because of the amount of time they spend around the loud sounds of music. Most musicians will spend time doing all of the following on a daily basis:

- Listening to their favorite musicians for inspiration, often at loud volumes in small rooms or through headphones or ear buds.
- Listening to their own music in the recording studio through headsets, typically at loud volume and for hours at a time.
- On stage playing loud and lively music in concert halls, small bars or clubs, and large concert venues. The noise on the stage in the middle of the music is deafening. The headsets some musicians wear may not mask all of the sound frequencies assaulting their ears.

- In the audience at very loud concerts, often sitting up by the stage near the speakers.
- Playing loud music in small, confined spaces during practice. The noise is amplified in small quarters, increasing the potential for hearing damage or tinnitus.

These situations are not limited to rock 'n' roll musicians. Musicians of all stripes can be found doing these very same things, either with or without knowledge of the damage they might be doing to their ears. This is why it is common for musicians to report ringing or other sound in the ears after they walk out of practice or get off stage from a concert. The sound might go away with time, but this is short-term tinnitus. Eventually, it could well become permanent.

It is very difficult for musicians to follow a lot of the advice given to others for protecting their ears. For example, it is commonly advised that you lower the volume in your ear buds or headphones when listening to portable music devices, such as iPods. It is also recommended that you limit the amount of time you spend listening through ear buds or headphones. This is difficult for musicians to do, as they need to listen to their own music in the recording studio, and they find inspiration in listening to their favorite artists.

The good news is there are some things musicians can do to protect their hearing as much as possible:

1. Have regular hearing tests so problems can be detected as early on as possible.

2. Keep the ears clean by washing with a warm wet washcloth. Earwax build-up can contribute to tinnitus.

3. Use ear plugs and other protective devices made for musicians. If you can mask at least some of the sound, you can take some of the risk for tinnitus away. This is, of course, not a guarantee that hearing loss or tinnitus will never become a problem.

4. Give the ears a break. Make it a point not to listen to music at loud volume when not in practice or in the studio. There is a lot you can learn by listening to rock 'n' roll at lower volumes.

That last tip is the best thing musicians can do for their ears. Give the ears a rest from the assault of noise and reduce the chances of developing tinnitus.

Tinnitus and the Rock Fan

Fans of rock 'n' roll music are at increased risk for developing tinnitus as well. They can even be at increased risk of hearing loss if they are in the habit of listening to their music at very high volume. Many concertgoers report hearing noises in their ears for an hour or two when they walk out of a concert. For those sitting too close to loud concert speakers, the tinnitus can be permanent and may come with partial or full hearing loss.

Listening to music at loud volumes for long periods of time through headphones or ear buds is also damaging to the ears. Music lovers who listen to music at loud volume in their bedrooms or other confined spaces are at high risk of suffering from tinnitus as well. Many rock lovers report hearing ringing or other noises right after listening to loud music, but it will go away within a few hours most of the time. With continued exposure, the loss can be permanent.

Some things that music lovers can do to protect their ears without giving up the rock include:

1. Turning the volume down. This is the simplest piece of advice, but it is the most effective piece of advice. Simply turn the volume down so the ears are not as traumatized by the noise.

2. Stopping the music at frequent points to give the ears a break. Whether listening to music through headphones or live in a bedroom or car, music lovers should turn the music off every hour or so to give the ears a break from the sound.

3. Taking breaks from loud concerts or night clubs and standing back from the stage and speakers. This may take a bit of the fun out of the event, but keeping full hearing without tinnitus is worth the sacrifice.

Music is one of the great joys of life for many, many people. But it can come with a price. There is no denying that there is a clear connection between tinnitus and rock 'n' roll and, really, most all forms of music, but there are things musicians and fans can do to limit the damage.

Tinnitus Lurks in Everyday Places

From the moment your head lifts from the pillow to the moment it drops back to the pillow at the end of the day, there are loud noises threatening your hearing ability. There are unexpected bursts of noise that could leave you with ringing ears. Your work or living environment may have continuous noise that strips away your hearing ability gradually over time.

Tinnitus lurks everywhere, every day, and for every one of us.

There are scores of things you could do on a daily basis to protect your ears and the ears of your children, but it basically comes down to being alert in everyday situations. To help you start thinking of ways to protect your hearing, consider 15 things you can do to protect your hearing in everyday life:

1. Cover your ears with protective headphones when doing lawn work with loud equipment. Snow and leaf blowers, tillers, lawn mowers, and other lawn and garden equipment can be extremely loud. If you are outside when these machines are in use or are using them yourself, cover your ears with headphones that block as much of the noise as possible.

2. When doing renovations on your home, landscaping outdoors, or working in a construction environment, protect your ears as much as possible. Wear protective headgear when it is safe and stay as far away as possible from loud tools being used by others. Chainsaws, bulldozers and other large equipment can be extremely damaging to the ears, especially when endured on a daily basis. If you cannot safely block all noise, use ear plugs to at least block part of the sound.

3. Wear ear plugs when you go hunting or visit the shooting range. The blast of gunfire can be damaging to the ears, especially if you stay at the range for a long period of time.

4. Talk with your children about the danger of loud noise. Instruct them to follow all of the tips on this list, plus others that relate directly to noises in their lives. No child is too young to start learning about protecting her ears.

5. Do not sit right by the speakers when at a concert or other event using a sound system or broadcasting loud music. If the sound is loud, it can damage your hearing. If the sound is mild, you never know when interference may send out a loud, shrill noise that can instantly damage your ears.

6. Acknowledge everyday noises that you may not be able to avoid all the time. For example, you may not want to wear ear plugs when taking your family to the amusement park, but you don't have to stand right under the loudest roller coaster while eating lunch. Think about your ears and do what you can to protect your hearing, even when complete avoidance is not possible.

7. Keep cheap moldable earplugs in your pocket when going to the movie theater. Sometimes the digital sound can lead to short-term tinnitus when you walk out of the theater. Moldable earplugs are cheap, compact enough to slip into your pocket or purse, and can provide instant filtering if the movie gets a bit too loud for your comfort. Bring some for young children as well.

8. If you have a home theater or watch movies in surround sound in your home, watch the volume. Even with regular television, turn it down! Consistent exposure to this loud noise can be damaging to your ear health, and that of everyone in your home.

9. If you go out to a nightclub where loud music is being played, take some time outside or in quieter areas of the club to give your ears a break. This should be done off and on throughout the night so your ears get a rest from the noise.

10. Always test the volume of toys that play music or make other sounds, especially if they will be played with by babies. Babies and toddlers often put toys up to their ears or lie down on their toys. If the toys are too loud, they could present a danger to young ears. If someone in your home already suffers from tinnitus, noisy toys could become annoying or frustrating.

11. If you show up at a restaurant that is featuring live entertainment, always ask to be seated away from the stage or speakers. You might not have the greatest view of the entertainment, but you will be able to talk more easily with your companions, and your ears won't be as offended.

12. Do not play loud music through headphones, or allow your children to play loud music through their headphones. Limit the amount of time children spend listening to mp3 players or having electronic devices read to them. These noises can be harmless to most people when the volume is controlled, but they can also be very damaging when used too often or when played too loud. Make sure teenagers understand the dangers involved when playing their iPods.

13. If you cannot talk to someone standing nearby without raising your voice, get out of that environment if possible. Whenever you have to raise your voice to be heard, you are in a loud environment that could be damaging to your hearing. Escape if it is at all possible.

14. If you experience ear ringing or other discomfort in the ears after a particular experience, know that that you need better protection the next time you go into that situation. This works for every experience you have in life. That ringing or discomfort is a cry of warning from your ears.

15. Rather than turning up the volume to drown out background noises, turn off the background noise. For example, don't turn up the living room television because a child is playing a video game too loudly down the hall. That video game is too loud, so turn it down and keep your volume down as well. When everyone starts upping the volume, all ears are potentially damaged.

Those are just some of the things you can do in everyday life to protect your hearing and the hearing of those you love. Think of the sources of noise in your everyday environment and ask yourself, what else can you be doing to reduce your risk of developing tinnitus or suffering from hearing loss?

Section 4:
Tinnitus Treatments

No. 1 Recommended Treatment:
Tinnitus Miracle

Product Review by Teresa J., Austin, Texas

If there is one commonly disputed claim in the medical industry today, it would be that there is no permanent cure for tinnitus. Many doctors resort to psychological and sound therapies to teach sufferers how to live with their conditions in as much comfort as possible, but they still maintain that there is no permanent solution to the problem. This has left thousands of sufferers around the world in search of a better solution – because they know there has to be one out there.

I know that desperate feeling of searching for something, anything at all, that will stop that constant ringing, buzzing or beeping in the ears. I lived with tinnitus for about 10 years and spent many nights staring at the ceiling of my dark bedroom, listening to the television or radio in the background, wondering when it would overtake the noise in my head. I woke up every morning thinking that there had to be a tinnitus treatment that would bring me tinnitus relief. Eventually, I found programs such as Tinnitus Miracle that finally showed me a way to the solution I knew had to be out there somewhere.

What is Tinnitus Miracle?

There are a few programs that claim to permanently get rid of the annoying noises caused by tinnitus and all of the other symptoms that come along with the noise. This even includes the more serious symptoms, such as dizziness and hearing loss. It has always been believed in the medical community that there is no way to permanently overcome these symptoms and get rid of tinnitus, but the Tinnitus Miracle ebook challenges that assumption.

Thousands of users have successfully used these programs, and Tinnitus Miracle is clearly one of the more popular options. The ebook is designed to walk sufferers of tinnitus through five steps that will ultimately end their agony with the annoying noises forever. The design of the book stands apart from others on the market because it is so easy to follow. Users simply follow from one easy step to the next and wait to see whether the noises and other symptoms go away.

What Does Tinnitus Miracle Claim?

So many products on the market today make big claims they cannot back up, but that has not been my experience with Tinnitus Miracle. Most users of this program feel some relief from their tinnitus within a week. For many people, this includes substantial changes for the better in their condition. While therapies with

a doctor can take months to take effect, this program can start the process of recovery in just days and bring complete relief in just two months.

This brings many people to assume that some type of expensive sound machine or medication must be behind the results, but that is not the case with Tinnitus Miracle. This program prides itself on ditching all the stereotypical tinnitus treatments, including:

- Medications
- Sound therapy
- Psychological therapy
- Surgery

Those treatments never helped me when I was suffering from the annoying buzz in my ears and they will not bring permanent relief to others either. That is because they are not designed for permanent relief. They are designed to teach sufferers to keep on suffering. I was no longer willing to suffer, and I know you aren't either.

The claims behind the Tinnitus Miracle may seem lofty, but they have been proven through years of research (which many other programs cannot claim) plus thousands of personal testimonies from people who have banished the hissing between the ears with this program.

Introducing Thomas Coleman

I am excited to "introduce" you to Thomas Coleman. He is the author of Tinnitus Miracle and a professional medical researcher. More important, he was a long-term sufferer of tinnitus before discovering the five-step process revealed in his ebook. This is important, because those who have never experienced tinnitus cannot possibly understand what it is like to suffer with it day in and day out.

The aggravation of the buzzing between the ears drove Thomas Coleman to find a solution to his problem, even though all the medical doctors told him there was no cure out there. It took him over 14 years to develop the program that he used to cure his own tinnitus, so he took it upon himself to pass that program on to other sufferers like me, you and thousands of others around the world.

What's the Catch?

There are catches to all programs that make bold claims, and the Tinnitus Miracle is no exception to the rule. The downside to this program is that you have to follow everything exactly as it is laid out in the ebook. The program is designed to be a holistic approach that tackles the most common causes of tinnitus. Miss or skip a step and you could sacrifice all or some of your results. Be prepared to commit fully if you go with this program.

When you order Tinnitus Miracle, you gain instant access to valuable information about your condition. You can place your order right now and start the program instantly. That means within the next week you could experience substantial relief from the ringing in your ears. If nothing else has worked for you, take this one last chance before giving up.

You can learn more about Tinnitus Miracle by going online to tinnitustreatmentoptions.com/tm

No. 2 Recommended Treatment:
Tinnitus Control

Product Review by Derek C., San Diego

How do you describe the noise going on inside your head? For me, it was an annoying buzz very similar to a muted bee that never went to sleep. Of course, the bee never sleeping meant *I* could never sleep.

Sound familiar?

There are stories like mine all over the world, as thousands of people suffer with long-term tinnitus. The reason so many people are suffering is clear: most believe that there is no permanent cure for their problem.

Because they believe there is no permanent cure, and that belief is often backed up by medical professionals who do not realize there are cures available, they suffer year after year needlessly. Then the lucky ones discover Tinnitus Control. I discovered it and I am excited to share it with you as well. Like all products, it has its pros and cons, so you will have to make up your own mind on whether it is worth a shot.

Tinnitus Control Pros

There are two big pros to using Tinnitus Control:

- It is a completely natural, holistic tinnitus treatment that presents no danger to your body.
- It is incredibly easy to use.

This is a holistic spray that you squirt under your tongue 1-3 times a day. You can take two squirts at a time and it can be repeated up to three times in a 24-hour period. There is nothing else to the product. Just squirt away and you will experience fast relief to the noises causing chaos between your ears.

What is really attractive about the product is that it is holistic. This simply means that it is a natural solution designed to treat "like with like." The basic idea of holistic medicine is that the body is presented with something known to create a symptom already being experienced, in order to get rid of that symptom. Holistic solutions are now being produced for everything from weight loss and headaches to tinnitus.

Holistic medicine often incorporates the emotional and spiritual as well as the physical, but Tinnitus Control obviously tackles only the physical. It is designed to get rid of the ringing in your ears quickly in a safe manner.

When the noise is driving you crazy, you simply squirt it away.

Tinnitus Control Cons

Obviously, this is not a substantial program designed to completely cure your tinnitus. There are programs out there like that, and some I have even had some success with, but this is not one of them. This product is designed for fast, but temporary, relief to the sounds associated with tinnitus. It doesn't claim to offer a complete cure, and it doesn't require any elaborate planning or maneuvering of your lifestyle.

The upside here is that you can use this spray for short-term or long-term tinnitus. If you still have hopes of getting rid of your tinnitus, then this is a product that can be helpful while you are searching for that permanent cure. It isn't the cure in itself, but it is a handy product that can bring substantial relief before the cure kicks in for you.

How to Properly Use Tinnitus Control

I have found this spray to be a lifesaver in particular situations, and you will probably find it to be a lifesaver as well. If you need temporary tinnitus relief so you can get through work without focusing more on the buzzing in your head than the meeting taking place around you, Tinnitus Control can come through for you. The same goes for getting through the day with the kids without feeling too sensitive to their excited screams or finding relief long enough to fall asleep at night.

Whenever you need a few hours of peace and quiet, you can depend on Tinnitus Control to come through for you.

Long-term relief? No.

Permanent relief? No.

Fast relief so you can get through the next few hours with maximum focus and peace of mind? Absolutely!

If you are having trouble reading this because of the annoyance inside your head, it may be time to try Tinnitus Control. The faster you visit their website and place your order, the faster you can spray away your tinnitus troubles.

Learn more about Tinnitus Control by going online to
tinnitustreatmentoptions.com/tc

No. 3 Recommended Treatment:
T-Gone Tinnitus Remedies

Product Review by Latisha T., Nebraska

D o you know what it is like to wake up in the middle of the night to a strange noise, only to remember that it is inside your own head? I have done this quite a few times in my life, so I know how frustrating it can be.

Fortunately, I also know how liberating it can be to find real solutions to the problem. I'm talking about solutions that make me look back at my many years of suffering with tinnitus as if it were a distant dream of someone else's life.

I still remember the discomfort of the condition, but I certainly do not miss it.

Once you discover the right solutions to your tinnitus problems, you will remember it without missing it as well. One product that I have found to be particularly useful is T-Gone Tinnitus Remedies. This actually refers to a series of tinnitus remedies produced by one company. There are a variety of formulas to select from, depending on the believed cause of your condition.

There are advantages and disadvantages to these remedies, just like all others. Consider this review carefully before deciding whether it might be worth a try for you.

T-Gone Tinnitus Remedies Advantages

T-Gone does not believe in producing one tinnitus remedy for everyone to use. Rather, they have created different holistic formulas for different types of tinnitus. The types of the condition are separated according to their believed causes. One person might be suffering from tinnitus brought on by a head injury, while someone else could be suffering from tinnitus brought on by stress. These people would take different formulas from T-Gone.

Another advantage to these remedies is that they are completely natural. They are based on holistic science and are not known to interact with any prescription medications. They may cancel themselves out when used with other holistic tinnitus treatments, but otherwise they are completely safe to take for all users.

Finally, I love T-Gone because they are so open with the information behind their products. You can find an ingredient list for all of their formulas on their website, complete with an explanation of why each ingredient was chosen for the formula. This is more information than you will find on most other products on the market today!

You can also find a variety of information about tinnitus in general when you read their website. You never take anything blind when you use T-Gone Tinnitus Remedies.

T-Gone Tinnitus Remedies Disadvantages

The biggest problem many people have with T-Gone remedies for tinnitus is that they don't always know what has caused their condition. Many people suffer from unexplained tinnitus, so they might have to make a good guess at which formula is right for them.

There are some products offered on the site that may be effective for those who are uncertain, but the actual holistic formulas are divided clearly by the cause of the problem. This can be a bit complicated for those who are not sure what has caused their condition.

It also takes some time for these remedies to work. This is not something that you spray under the tongue and experience fast relief from. The recommended length of treatment is 90 days, but many users will have to take it for longer periods of time to completely get rid of their tinnitus. It is a gradual process, but one that will pay off for many in the end.

Should You Give It a Try?

If you have spent much of your life suffering in silence because you thought there was no way to get rid of your tinnitus, then T-Gone Tinnitus Remedies could be the last product you have to try. Since they separate their remedies according to the type of tinnitus you are experiencing, you don't have to second guess whether it will work with your problem. You can read the extensive information on the website regarding your specific cause of the condition to determine whether you trust T-Gone or not.

At the end of the day, they offer a 100% money back guarantee, so you aren't really risking anything by giving it a try. Start out with a 90-day supply of the formula geared to your cause of tinnitus and see what happens. If the progress is too slow going for you or you don't feel you are making any progress, then you can send it back and get a refund. Nothing is lost if nothing is gained.

Learn more about T-Gone Tinnitus Remedies by going online to tinnitustreatmentoptions.com/tgtr

Five More Effective Tinnitus Treatment Options

Tinnitus can interfere with the daily lives of sufferers, but with the right treatment program it can be made bearable. Some treatment options are designed to teach sufferers how to cope with their disorder, while other treatments directly combat common symptoms of the disorder to bring as much relief as possible. Most sufferers benefit from mixing and matching the following tinnitus treatment options to create an individualized treatment program.

Talk Therapy

Many people do not see the value in talk therapy as a form of tinnitus treatment, but it can actually be very effective for long-term sufferers. Because the condition never goes away or takes years to go away, most sufferers have to learn how to accept their condition and move on with their lives. They have to learn how to live with it, because the only other option is to stop living.

Talk therapy is effective because it gives sufferers an outlet where they can discuss how they are feeling and how they are dealing with the condition. They are able to discuss how other forms of tinnitus treatment are working (or not working) and can come to grips with their emotions associated with the condition.

Talk therapy doesn't have to involve a professional all the time. Many sufferers benefit from having friends and relatives they can turn to when they are having a difficult time or are struggling with particularly hard days with the condition. Some may even find refuge with online tinnitus support groups. Just having that outlet to talk it through can make living with the condition much easier.

Cognitive Behavior Therapy

This is different from talk therapy in that it involves a lot of action. Someone going through cognitive behavior therapy for a phobia may be exposed directly to the source of their phobia, but it is a bit different for those suffering with tinnitus. The therapy involves direct exposure to different situations where the tinnitus might be at its worst. They learn to react differently to the condition, so it doesn't seem as bad in their minds.

This is all about playing mind games, but it is a very effective treatment for tinnitus. Sufferers learn new ways of handling their condition in the moment, so they start to think about it and process it in a new way. This will not make the condition go away, but it will make the condition much easier to cope with long term.

This form of therapy may make the difference between someone learning to deal with the condition in their social lives or at work and someone feeling unable to interact with others and continue working. Minor cases may not affect sufferers to this extent, but for those with more severe cases, it is a reality.

Noise Generators/Machines

Machines that create white noise and generators that create sounds from the natural environment can be effective forms of tinnitus treatment. These machines are used to create a new noise in the sufferer's background, which will hopefully drown out and quiet down the sound being produced from the tinnitus. Again, this does nothing to completely get rid of tinnitus. It is just another way to control the condition, especially when the sufferer is trying to relax or fall asleep.

Medication

Some medications can be used as a treatment for tinnitus, but there are no medications that will completely cure the problem. Here is a quick rundown on some of the more prominent medications used for the condition today:

- Niacin – there is currently no scientific proof that this works, but some claim it does.
- Gabapentin – can help reduce the severity of the noise, but it does not work for everyone.
- Acamprosate – one of the more promising options, but studies are still being conducted.
- Zinc – effective only if the body is low on zinc.

The last two medications on this list are probably the most effective options, though zinc works only if your body has a zinc deficit. If low zinc levels are not a factor in the cause of the tinnitus, it should not be supplemented.

Lifestyle Adjustments

This is what many tinnitus treatments come down to in the end. Sufferers hope that the condition will go away, but until that happens they have no choice but to adjust their lifestyle to decrease their sensitivity to the condition. This may be done through some form of therapy, or it can simply be avoiding places that have high noise levels.

Changing your lifestyle because of tinnitus is not a pleasant experience, but it makes life much easier for those suffering from the condition long term or permanently.

For more on lifestyle changes, see the chapter on "Changing Your Lifestyle to Prevent Tinnitus" (page 81).

Natural Strategies for Tinnitus Relief

When tinnitus doesn't go away within a few weeks and the condition stretches out into months or years, the biggest concern is what quality of life the sufferer will be able to have.

This is not an easy to condition to live with the rest of your life, but there are some ways to find tinnitus relief. Some people can use these natural strategies to make their tinnitus bearable, while others will get moderate relief that makes life a little better than it otherwise might be.

How much relief could these tinnitus remedies bring? You will never know until you start giving some of them a try. It is best to try them one at a time so you can tell what is bringing tinnitus relief and what is not working for you. What works for someone else won't necessarily work for you, and vice versa. You have to go through your options with a trial-and-error approach to find a treatment plan that makes your life easier.

Things to Avoid

Tinnitus relief is often gained to varying extents when the following items are avoided:

- Cigarette smoke
- Alcohol
- Salt
- Caffeine
- Simple sugars
- Saturated fats
- Trans fats
- Loud noise
- Aspirin

Cigarette smoke probably increases tinnitus because it is an irritant to the body. So many things are drastically improved when smoking is stopped, and tinnitus is at the top of that list.

This doesn't mean just not smoking yourself. It means staying away from others when they are smoking and in environments full of smoke as well. For example, someone with tinnitus may experience worse symptoms when sitting at a poker game where everyone is smoking, even if they are not smoking themselves.

Salt has a negative effect on tinnitus because it increases blood pressure, which can restrict blood flow to the ears. Sugars affect the auditory system, which can negatively affect hearing (and tinnitus). Unhealthy fats negatively affect cholesterol, which can have a negative effect on tinnitus.

Exposure to loud noise can make tinnitus worse and may even lead to hearing loss, which is a component in many cases of permanent tinnitus.

Avoiding these things will not cure tinnitus, but can lead to significant tinnitus relief so it is much easier to live with in the long term.

Things to Try

There are a few supplements that also can bring some tinnitus relief, including:

- Melatonin
- Gingko Biloba
- Niacin

Melatonin is designed to regulate your natural sleep/wake cycle, which can help those suffering from sleep deprivation caused by tinnitus. Many people have trouble falling asleep or staying asleep because of the ringing in their ears. Melatonin can help them overcome these problems, but it works best when combined with some other natural tinnitus relief strategies:

- Going to sleep on a routine schedule
- Setting up a comfortable sleep environment
- Using light background noise to minimize the noise inside the head.

Gingko biloba and niacin are also claimed to work effectively against tinnitus, but they do not work for everyone. There is no substantial research to show that niacin really works, and neither of these supplements is guaranteed to work for everyone.

Control Blood Pressure

High blood pressure, also known as hypertension, can cause a pulsating sensation or noise that resembles a pulsing pattern.

This comes from the blood pulsing through the interior arteries, which are restricted as a result of the hypertension. This means less blood is going to the ears, yet the blood is being pumped extra hard in an attempt to get it there. This intensifies tinnitus and can even cause pulsatile tinnitus.

Pump Up the (Background) Volume

Turning on some form of light background noise can help distract from or drown out the noise being caused by the tinnitus. This is one of the best ways to get tinnitus relief, since it is one of the few treatment options that work on virtually all sufferers. It may seem like adding to the noise would only complicate the problem, but many people find that the tinnitus noise is soft enough that they can blur it at least a little with noise from a television, radio, or white noise machine.

Biofeedback

Biofeedback trains the body and mind to connect in a new way. When it is used effectively, patients are taught how to react to stress and tension so it doesn't have as much negative impact on their lives. For tinnitus, biofeedback can be used to change the way the sufferer reacts to tinnitus. Many people do get tinnitus relief when biofeedback is applied by a professional.

Another Natural Strategy:
Deep Breathing Exercises

Deep breathing exercises can be very powerful when suffering from long-term tinnitus. If you find yourself depressed and unable to cope with daily life, you can use these exercises to improve your mood and overcome irritability. You can also use these exercises to control stress and relieve physical and mental tension, which may aggravate your tinnitus.

Deep breathing exercises are often prescribed to those suffering from anxiety disorders and many other psychological conditions. Because anxiety, increased stress, mood swings, and depression are common to long-term sufferers of tinnitus, they can become a part of the long-term strategy for coping with this disorder.

Following are a few deep breathing techniques that can be useful in daily life. They will give you a foundation of knowledge that can be used in a variety of everyday situations. Use this knowledge to come up with creative ways to use deep breathing in your own daily world.

Corpse Breathing

Do this when you have a bit of time to invest, or when you are feeling particularly down and don't feel like doing anything else. Lie on your back in the floor with your arms relaxed at your sides and your legs relaxed straight out on the floor. (This exercise is sometimes referred to as "corpse breathing" because the position you are in on the floor resembles that of a corpse.) Take a couple of normal breaths and notice what part of your body is rising and falling as you inhale and exhale. The areas of potential movement are in the chest, stomach, and abdomen.

If you feel most of the rise and fall in your stomach and abdomen, you are breathing deeply. Take time to focus on that breathing. Inhale and feel your chest rise, and focus on forcing your stomach and abdomen to rise as well. Exhale deeply, slowly forcing all air out so you can inhale deeply again.

If you feel most of the rise and fall in your chest, your breathing is quite shallow. The air is not being pulled and pushed all the way down into your abdomen, which is where it goes with healthy deep breathing. Take time to focus on breathing deeply, with the stomach and abdomen rising right along with the chest.

Just lying on the floor, closing your eyes, and focusing on drawing deep breaths while feeling the air enter and leave your body can be very soothing. You will learn how to take deeper breaths to bring more oxygen to the brain. This will help with your sense of overall well-being, will help improve focus and attention, and will give you some energy to tackle the day.

Use what you learn about breathing deeply from this exercise for all of the other exercises listed below. This is the deep breathing that you want to perform when you just need to relax and take an edge off.

5-Minute Deep Breathing

If you have just 5 minutes, you can use deep breathing to pump up your spirit and refresh your mind. You need a quiet space where you can get into a comfortable position, close your eyes, and focus on your breathing without distraction. If possible, cutting the lights and turning off the television will help.

This exercise needs to be sustained for 5 minutes, so set a timer if possible. This way, you don't have to open your eyes and break concentration just to check how much time is remaining.

Once comfortable, close your eyes and focus on deepening your breathing just as you did in the exercise above. The more you practice this, the easier it will be to get into a comfortable position and start breathing deeper. With each breath, go deeper and deeper, trying to feel that expansion all the way down to your abdomen.

Keep doing this for 5 minutes without breaking concentration. If you start to feel your mind wander to other things, simply refocus on your breathing. Focus on how the air feels entering and leaving your body. Focus on oxygen entering the brain and boosting your well-being.

After 5 minutes, open your eyes and ease back into your day. You should feel different if you were able to concentrate only on breathing and relax for the entire 5 minutes.

Simple Deep Breathing Exercises

You can create a variety of deep breathing exercises to improve your mood and release stress just by combining the deep breathing pattern you have already learned and the concepts of holding your breath and contracting your hands or legs.

Take a couple of deep breaths right now, and on the second inhale hold the breath for just a few seconds before slowly releasing your breath. This is the concept of holding your breath.

Take a couple of more deep breaths, but this time put your hands out in front of your body or over your head. On the second inhale, hold the breath and squeeze your hands together. Release your hands and slowly exhale. This is the concept of creating tension in your hands.

Now, you can use these simple breathing strategies in any situation needed. While sitting at your desk at work and fighting to stay focused and alert, you can stretch your arms out over the desk, take a few deep breaths while holding the inhale and squeezing your hands. At home, you can spend time just lying on the couch or bed breathing deeply rather than staring at the walls depressed.

Deep Breathing and Tinnitus

Remember that these deep breathing strategies are great for anyone suffering from depression, anxiety, overwhelming stress, and many other psychological disorders. How they might help your tinnitus remains to be seen. You will have to experiment with different settings, body positions, and types of breathing to determine what soothes your tinnitus, or at least does not intensify the sound.

Deep breathing is completely natural and without risk, so it can be used with all other forms of tinnitus treatment. For example, if you are using background noise as a method of masking your tinnitus for improved concentration at work, you could also use deep breathing exercises to calm the mind, release tension and enhance concentration further.

Changing Your Lifestyle to Prevent Tinnitus

Is it possible to prevent tinnitus just by controlling your lifestyle? In the case of the more rare pulsatile tinnitus, this is not typically possible. But for most other forms of tinnitus, it is possible for most people.

If you understand some of the more common causes of tinnitus, you will see exactly what you need to do on a daily basis to limit your risk of developing the disorder. This chapter will introduce you to these more common causes while telling you easy ways to live a healthy life with lower risks of tinnitus.

Don't Take Your Ears for Granted

This is the best piece of advice you will ever get on protecting yourself from tinnitus. Most people never think about protecting their ears until they experience tinnitus for the first time. You can possibly avoid it from ever setting in if you take some precautions in your daily life.

How do you protect your ears? You simply use caution when around any source of loud noise. If you go to a concert, do not sit right next to the speakers. The best seats for a visual view may be right on the speakers, but that view is not worth risking a bout of tinnitus. In some cases, the noise from those speakers will cause permanent tinnitus. Those speakers could also leave you with hearing loss.

Watch the volume when playing music or listening to audio programs through headphones or ear buds as well. You can learn a lot by listening to lead singer of the rock group The Who, Pete Townshend. He has been very open with the public regarding his hearing loss and tinnitus, which was originally assumed to be the result of so many hours spent playing with the band in clubs and practicing in small studios.

Townshend went public in 2006 with his belief that listening to music through headphones in the studio was what caused his tinnitus. He also made a point in one interview that his ears never rang after concerts unless the band played in small venues. You can turn this information into clear advice on protecting your own ears:

- Avoid loud concerts in smaller venues.
- Watch the volume when listening through headphones.
- Limit the number of hours spent listening to headphones each day.

Loud noise can also be found in some industrial work settings or even just walking down a busy urban street at times. Even a short-term burst of very loud sound can lead to tinnitus, hearing loss, or both.

Healthy Waistline, Healthy Ears

Most people think of a well-balanced diet and exercise as the recipe for staying thin and looking their best in a bathing suit, but diet and exercise are actually some of the best ways to lower your risk of developing tinnitus. Studies are showing that the irregular and forceful blood circulation that comes along with cardiovascular disease is a contributing factor to the experience of tinnitus for some patients.

This means you can reduce your chance of experiencing tinnitus by protecting your heart. How do you protect your heart? You eat nutrient-dense foods that do not contain a lot of artery-clogging saturated fat. You also exercise so your body burns off far more calories than it stores away as fat each day. This will protect your heart from disease, which in turn protects your ears from tinnitus.

Regular Check-Ups

It is important to get yearly physicals with a medical doctor and biannual check-ups with a dentist. There are some medical conditions that cause tinnitus as a symptom. Some dental problems can also cause tinnitus, including problems with the alignment of the jaw. If you receive regular check-ups you are more likely to know that you have a medical condition or dental problem that leaves you at higher risk for tinnitus. The rest of your lifestyle choices become far more important if you have this risk.

If you do have a condition that leaves you at risk for tinnitus, you can treat the condition in order to lower that risk. For example, if you have a thyroid problem that could cause tinnitus, you should take medication to correct the thyroid problem. This will improve your overall health while leaving you less vulnerable to the pain of tinnitus.

Tinnitus can also be caused by excessive build-up of wax in the ears. A medical doctor will check your ears when you go in for a physical, so these smaller risks will be eliminated.

If you are very concerned with your risk of developing tinnitus, make sure to ask your doctor about all medications that are prescribed. There are some medications that may leave you vulnerable to tinnitus, but you can ask your doctor to prescribe something that does not include tinnitus as a potential side effect.

Protection from Injury

Some cases of tinnitus are caused by injury to the neck or head. In many cases this type of injury cannot be avoided, but for others the injury comes as a direct result of lifestyle choices. If you do any type of sport or hobby that entails traveling at high speeds or falling from heights, you risk an injury that could lead to tinnitus.

You don't want to stop living your life or enjoying your hobbies out of fear. You should, however, protect yourself in case of an accident. This may mean wearing a helmet while riding four wheelers or while racing a motorcycle. It may mean wearing protective equipment when you go rock climbing. If there is protective equipment available for your sport, wear it religiously.

There may never be a way to completely protect yourself from tinnitus. Many people never know for sure what caused their tinnitus, especially if it goes away after a short period of time. But if you are willing to make some lifestyle changes to protect your body from the most common causes of the disorder, you can at least reduce your chances of experiencing tinnitus in the future.

Introduction to Tinnitus Retraining Therapy

There are currently no permanent cures for tinnitus, but tinnitus retraining therapy is one treatment that may come very close for many sufferers. Although many people learn to live with tinnitus through talk therapy and cognitive behavioral therapy, this newer form of therapy is in the discipline of neuroscience. Yet, the goal of all three therapies is to change the way sufferers think about and approach their tinnitus conditions.

It may be difficult for some people to find qualified medical professionals to administer tinnitus retraining therapy properly, but those who can find treatment have yet another effective option for living comfortably with tinnitus.

What is Tinnitus Retraining Therapy?

Tinnitus retraining therapy, or TRT, is a neurologically-based approach that combines noise therapy with talk therapy. Patients are trained to understand all elements of tinnitus as well as coping mechanisms for dealing with condition. They are also treated with special sound therapy that delivers lower levels of broadband noise to the ears. In most cases, this is simply in the form of varying background noises that can effectively cover the sounds being created by the tinnitus.

Through the use of the background noise and educational therapies that teach critical skills to override the tinnitus noises, it is believed that patients can learn to disregard their tinnitus. This means they continue living with the condition, but in most cases they forget that the sound is there. They simply learn to tune it out and focus on other aspects of their life and their surroundings.

One element of tinnitus retraining therapy is to teach patients a new way of thinking about their condition and responding to the noise associated with their conditions. Most people have a very negative experience suffering with tinnitus, so they think of their noises in a very negative fashion. This is entirely understandable, but it makes living with the condition more difficult. Because many people have no choice but to live with the noises inside their heads long term or even the rest of their lives, it is to their benefit to learn to look at the noise in a more favorable light.

Eventually, patients transition from losing the negativity associated with their condition to not thinking much about their condition at all. This is the goal of tinnitus retraining therapy: to get patients to a point of acceptance where they do not focus on their tinnitus most of the time. It is always there, but if they learn to accept it and then to turn their minds away from it, daily life can become a lot more tolerable. For some, it may even become almost normal again.

The Nature of Tinnitus Retraining Therapy

It is important for tinnitus patients to understand that they have to fully invest their minds in this type of therapy if it is to be successful. If someone believes that it cannot work or does not fully invest herself in learning the strategies taught by medical professionals, then chances are high that relief from tinnitus will not be achieved.

Those who get the most from tinnitus retraining therapy are those who believe that it can work, listen to everything that they are taught, and actively put those new lessons into practice in their daily life. This is the same type of dedication that is needed to get effective results from talk therapy or cognitive behavioral therapy. The difference is that TRT combines sound therapy with talk therapy. The strategies used to turn the thoughts in a positive direction may also be different, depending on the therapist being consulted and the form of therapy embraced.

Is TRT a Cure?

Many claim that TRT is a complete cure, because it can redirect the brain so that the symptoms of the condition are no longer picked up on a daily basis. It is true that some people may find this level of relief, but it isn't always seen as a complete cure of the condition. It is more like a redirection of the mind that changes the way the condition is perceived by the brain. Yet, for some it may feel like a complete recovery from tinnitus.

Section 5: Related Diseases

Pulsatile Tinnitus Linked to Life-Threatening Diseases

Tinnitus is a medical condition that thousands of people all around the world suffer from. Although it usually is characterized by a ringing in the ears, a variety of noises or sounds can occur. Some may hear a beeping sound while others hear chirping. Pulsatile tinnitus is a rare form of the condition that is characterized by a pulsating sound or sensation.

Just like any other type of tinnitus, pulsatile tinnitus can be short lived or it can be a permanent condition. In some it may be a minor annoyance while in others it is a severe medical condition that interferes with daily life. Some people may experience the pulsating sensation off and on over a period of time, while it may be a continuous experience for others.

What Is Pulsatile Tinnitus?

Tinnitus is most often caused by extremely loud noise or trauma to the head or neck that damages the auditory system in some manner. It may sometimes be accompanied by a hearing loss in one or both ears, but this isn't always the case.

Pulsatile tinnitus also can be caused by trauma to the head or neck, but it can just as easily be caused by high blood pressure, brain tumors or a variety of serious medical conditions. This connection to life-threatening diseases or conditions makes this form of tinnitus the most serious.

The pulsing sensation felt with this condition is in sync with the rhythm of the heartbeat. Every time the heart beats, there is a pulsation or noise in the ears or head. This can be continuous or it may come and go, depending on the exact cause and nature of the individual condition. The basic cause for this form of tinnitus is disruption or restriction in blood flow through the neck and/or head.

The good news is that not many people have to suffer with this form of tinnitus. It is the most unusual diagnosis of all tinnitus cases, affecting roughly 3% of all tinnitus sufferers. The bad news is that it can be a little more difficult to treat than other forms of tinnitus and can have serious consequences. For example, if left untreated, it could lead to stroke. Because it also could be connected to a brain tumor or extreme hypertension, it must be diagnosed and treated by a medical professional as quickly as possible.

Treating Pulsatile Tinnitus

Many medical professionals recommend tinnitus retraining therapy as the best form of treatment for pulsatile tinnitus. This is a unique form of therapy that teaches the brain not to pay attention to the sounds presented by the tinnitus. This is done through the use of background sounds with a sound device as well as through therapy sessions that train sufferers how to effectively move beyond the noise and enjoy an active life.

This form of therapy has actually proven to be quite successful for many tinnitus sufferers, but for those with pulsatile tinnitus the treatment doesn't end there.

In many cases there is a more serious cause for the tinnitus that must be treated as well. Treating the actual noises of tinnitus becomes a secondary concern to fixing the hypertension, tumor or other serious medical issue causing the tinnitus. Pulsatile tinnitus is thus seen as a symptom in these cases, rather than the actual condition to be contended with.

Do You Have Pulsatile Tinnitus?

Many people will suffer with pulsatile tinnitus for a long time before realizing that there is an actual medical condition that fits what they are experiencing.

In some cases, they will learn that they are suffering from a medical condition only when other symptoms of the bigger medical cause start to present themselves.

That is a shame, because they could have experienced faster relief from their condition and gotten treatment for any serious medical conditions if they would have seen a doctor about their symptoms earlier on.

Anyone suffering from a pulsing sensation or noise that seems to keep a beat with their heart should see a medical professional immediately. This is a form of tinnitus that should not be ignored or downplayed.

Hyperacusis: A Patient's Guide

Pay attention to the sounds in your natural environment right now. There might be a television or radio playing in the background. You might be able to hear other people talking in the next room or down the hallway. There may be footfall somewhere near, birds chirping outside the window, or a child banging a basketball on the pavement just feet from where you are sitting.

Most people hear all of these environmental sounds on a routine basis and they barely register on the brain, but someone suffering from hyperacusis will have a very different reaction to those same sounds.

Hyperacusis is a medical condition in which the sufferer has an extreme sensitivity to sounds. Different patients can be more sensitive to sounds of a different frequency, and some cases are more severe than others. Yet, they all hear everyday noises very different from the rest of the world. They hear these sounds at an amplified volume and it is an extreme agitation, or sometimes a source of pain.

Signs of Hyperacusis

Most people with hyperacusis simply find certain types of sounds annoying or painful. In mild cases, they may hear sounds of certain frequencies and feel a deep sense of annoyance and agitation. In more severe cases, they may experience real pain when they hear noises of a certain frequency. Some can tolerate louder noises than others, so the exact experience differs from one sufferer to the next.

Most loved ones discover that something is wrong when they notice someone they care about cannot tolerate noise as others do. They may notice a child with hyperacusis putting their hands over their ears and crying when other children screech and play excitedly nearby. They may notice that an adult gets extremely annoyed when an emergency vehicle goes by with the sirens blaring.

Any type of intolerance of noise can be a sign of hyperacusis, but it doesn't necessarily mean a diagnosis is a sure thing. A medical professional has to get involved for an official diagnosis and a determination of potential causes.

Hyperacusis and Tinnitus

Tinnitus is known as the medical condition that causes ringing in the ears, although it can include a variety of sounds besides ringing. It is often believed that tinnitus and hyperacusis are related, but they don't always go hand-in-hand. Some people will experience both of these conditions together, but many others experience only one or the other.

Some of the treatments for hyperacusis will also treat tinnitus, and vice versa. The conditions are clearly related and are often caused by the same experiences. For example, most cases of tinnitus are caused by exposure to loud noise or trauma to the head or neck. Those happen to be common causes of hyperacusis as well.

Treatment for Hyperacusis

Therapy is typically used to help people suffering from hyperacusis. Talk therapy can be used to help sufferers handle everyday life with extreme sensitivity to sound, but most patients will also undergo therapies designed to desensitize them to the sounds that bother them most.

These therapies use exposure to a variety of sounds of differing frequencies in order to get the sufferers more used to tolerating a variety of sounds. This can take some time, so patients have to invest themselves fully and have patience throughout the process.

There are different sound machines and devices that can be used for desensitization therapy, but bilateral broadband signal generators are a popular option today. These devices are used by many medical professionals offering therapy for sufferers of this medical condition.

Epilog

One of the messages I have tried to convey in this book is how important it is to take care of your ears, your hearing. So few people do. And often the damage is done before they understand just how important our ears are. That's a shame.

Let me repeat the beginning of the chapter "Tinnitus Lurks in Everyday Places" (page 53):

> From the moment your head lifts from the pillow to the moment it drops back to the pillow at the end of the day, there are loud noises threatening your hearing ability. There are unexpected bursts of noise that could leave you with ringing ears. Your work or living environment may have continuous noise that strips away your hearing ability gradually over time.
>
> *Tinnitus lurks everywhere, every day, and for every one of us.*

We teach our children to brush their teeth. We warn them against looking directly into the sun, and to protect their skin from too much exposure to the sun. We tell them to be sure to look both ways before crossing the street. The list goes on and on.

But how many of us teach our children how to protect their ears? Hearing is the most neglected of the senses, and, unfortunately, it's also one of the most fragile.

As chronicled in the Foreword, I have lived with tinnitus for most of my life. Despite all the tests I underwent over the years, the medical profession has never been able to tell me why, at age 10, I suddenly developed a high-pitched whine in my ears that has never stopped. Fortunately, my tinnitus has been a relatively mild case, and I have learned to live with it.

At age 14 I began working summers for my father, who was a carpenter. I did my ears no favor by not wearing any protection whenever I operated power saws, sanders, lathes and other noisy equipment. I can't say all that noise had an immediate impact on my tinnitus, but it certainly didn't help anything. My father, who worked unprotected around such noise year around for decades, lost most of his hearing by the time he was in his early 60s.

I was first diagnosed with a "mild" hearing loss when I was in my mid-30s, long after I had ceased working for Dad. Whether my tinnitus contributed to my hearing loss is another question medical science cannot answer. But it is possible it did. My noisy summers working for my father also might have played a role.

At any rate, my hearing has continued to decline over the years. At this writing, I am 72. To give you some idea of the state of my hearing today, I can tell you that I usually have to ask people, sometimes more than once, and especially women, to repeat whatever it is they have said to me.

I have spent thousands of dollars on hearing aids, mostly to no avail. It's not that these devices do not amplify the sound that is coming into my ears (and that includes *all* sounds, not just the voices you want to hear, so that a conversation while wearing hearing aids in a noisy restaurant, for example, is no better for me than a conversation without them).

The main problem with hearing aids, for me and others as well, is that they make sounds, including your own voice, seem *unnatural*. The feeling that I have when I stuff these little devices into my ears is eerily like the feeling I described in the Foreword when my ears started ringing for the first time when I was 10 years old. I repeat that description here:

> It was as if I was in a dream. Nothing seemed quite real. If I had been an adult, I might have said that it almost resembled an out-of-body experience, or that I was having a panic attack. My voice sounded strange to me, remote, and I seemed to have no control over what I was saying. My mother's voice seemed to be coming through a heavy veil I could not see.

But the loss of hearing has had a far greater impact on my life than the inconvenience of having to ask people to repeat themselves, or the uncomfortable feeling that wearing hearing aids gives me, as troublesome as those things are.

Much more important to me is that my hearing loss has robbed me, and I'm sure many others as well, of some of the joys of life.

I go to a movie, but I cannot really discuss it afterwards because there was so much of it I missed.

I sit at a holiday table with the people I love, and I watch them talk and laugh and tell stories, but most often I don't know what they are saying.

I take a walk in a beautiful wood, but I cannot hear the birds sing.

A small grandchild lays her hand on mine and says something to me in her tiny voice. I do not ask her to repeat. I give her a hug and tell her I love her. I hope she understands.

And so, what has happened is that I have shrunk my world. If at all possible, I avoid parties and get-togethers of one sort and another. I go to movies less often, and to stage plays not at all.

My wife answers the phone. If I am home alone, the caller will have to leave a message. Any business that must be done over the phone also is handled for me by my wife.

I try never to have to ride with someone in a car. In a car the only thing I can hear is the roar of the highway.

I stay away from the occasional person who makes fun of my hearing loss. (Yes, there are people who will mock you for your hearing handicap. Sad but true.)

I say all these things not to make you feel sorry for me, and not because I am feeling sorry for myself. Quite the contrary. I have a very good life, much to live for and much to be thankful for.

Rather, I say these things because I want you to understand what the consequences could be – for you and for those you love – if you do not take care of your ears.

If you already are suffering from tinnitus, try one of the tinnitus treatment options discussed in this book. If a loved one is a tinnitus victim, pass this book along to her or him.

See a doctor, and get your hearing checked regularly.

And always, always, protect your ears. You lose so much more than your hearing if you don't.

Grab all of life that you can – it is full of love and music and all things incredible.

Listen to the birds sing. – *Dave Carmichael, 2012*

Addendum

Pine-Bark Extract Shows Promise
as a Natural Tinnitus Relief

A recent study indicates that a pine bark extract has promise as a natural remedy for tinnitus. The extract apparently works by improving blood flow in the inner ear, thereby reducing or eliminating one of the chief causes of tinnitus.

In a study conducted by the Chieti-Pescara University in Italy, researchers took 82 patients between the ages of 35 and 55 with mild to moderate tinnitus in only one ear and studied them for one month. Their tinnitus was caused by restricted blood supply to the inner ear.

The patients were divided into three groups. Group A consisted of 24 patients who took 150 mg a day of the pine-bark extract. Group B had 34 patients who took 100 mg a day. A control group had 24 patients who did not take the extract.

After four weeks of treatment with pine bark, inner-ear blood-flow velocities to the affected ears rose significantly. The results indicated that the extract improved circulation and reduced tinnitus. Researchers said the results suggest the pine-bark extract might work as a treatment for the condition.

The study looked at how pine bark affected the symptoms of tinnitus. Patients rated their symptoms from "zero" (low intensity symptoms) to 15 (constant and severe symptoms). Prior to the study, the patients' average rating was 8.8. After the study, the average had dropped to 5.2 in the lower-dose group and 3.3 in the higher-dose group. There were no significant changes in the rating for the control group.

The study was published in Panminerva Medica, a journal on internal medicine. The extract used was pycnogenol (pic-noj-en-all), an antioxidant plant extract derived from the bark of the French maritime pine tree.

17001525R10059

Made in the USA
Lexington, KY
25 August 2012